Mosby's
Veterinary
PDQ

Veterinary Facts at Hand
Practical • Detailed • Quick

Inside you will find:

- Surgical Nursing Procedures
- Animal Care Techniques
- Common Drugs
- Common Diseases
- Lab Tests
- Imaging Techniques
- Parasite Identification
- Urine Sediment
- Dentistry Procedures
- Surgical and Dental Instruments

plus much more.

ELSEVIER

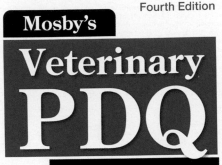

Fourth Edition

Mosby's Veterinary PDQ

Veterinary Facts at Hand
Practical • Detailed • Quick

Consultant
Kristin Holtgrew-Bohling, DVM

ELSEVIER

MOSBY'S VETERINARY PDQ,
FOURTH EDITION

ISBN: 978-0-323-88149-4

Notice

Practitioners and researchers must always rely on their own
experience and knowledge in evaluating and using any information,
methods, compounds or experiments described herein. Because of
rapid advances in the medical sciences, in particular, independent
verification of diagnoses and drug dosages should be made. To the
fullest extent of the law, no responsibility is assumed by Elsevier,
authors, editors or contributors for any injury and/or damage to
persons or property as a matter of products liability, negligence or
otherwise, or from any use or operation of any methods, products,
instructions, or ideas contained in the material herein.

Previous editions copyrighted 2019, 2014, 2009.

Content Strategist: Melissa Rawe
Director, Content Development: Laurie Gower
Senior Content Development Specialist: Aparajita Basu
Publishing Services Manager: Deepthi Unni
Senior Project Manager: Kamatchi Madhavan
Design Direction: Ryan Cook

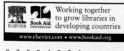

Working together
to grow libraries in
developing countries

www.elsevier.com • www.bookaid.org

Printed in China

Last digit is the print number: 9 8 7 6 5 4 3 2 1

ANATOMICAL PLANES OF REFERENCE[14,35]

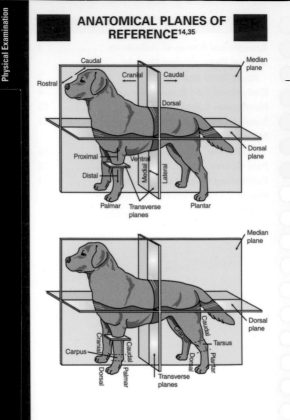

NORMAL PHYSIOLOGICAL DATA IN ADULT DOGS AND CATS

	Heart Rate (Beats/Min)	Respiratory Rate (Breaths/Min)	Rectal Temperature (°C)	Rectal Temperature (°F)
Dogs	70–160	8–20	37.5°C–39.0°C	99.5°F–102.2°F
Cats	150–210	8–30	38°C–39°C	100.4°F–102.2°F

BODY CONDITION SCORING SYSTEM

Body Condition Scoring System (Canine)[14]

Too Thin

BCS 1
- Ribs, lumbar vertebrae, pelvic bones, and all bony prominences evident from a distance
- No discernible body fat
- Obvious loss of muscle mass

BCS 2
- Ribs, lumbar vertebrae, and pelvic bones easily visible
- No palpable fat
- Some bony prominences visible from a distance
- Minimal loss of muscle mass

BCS 3
- Ribs easily palpable and may be visible with no palpable fat
- Tops of lumber vertebrae visible, pelvic bones becoming prominent
- Obvious waist and abdominal tuck

BCS 4

- Ribs easily palpable with minimal fat covering
- Waist easily noted when viewed from above
- Abdominal tuck evident

Ideal

BCS 5

- Ribs palpable without excess fat covering
- Waist observed behind ribs when viewed from above
- Abdomen tucked up when viewed from side

Overweight

BCS 6

- Ribs palpable with slight excess of fat covering
- Waist is discernible when viewed from above but is not prominent
- Abdominal tuck apparent

Continued

Body Condition Scoring System (Canine)[14]

BCS 7

- Ribs palpable with difficulty, heavy fat cover
- Noticeable fat deposits over lumbar area and base of tail
- Waist absent or barely visible
- Abdominal tuck may be absent

BCS 8

- Ribs not palpable under very heavy fat cover or palpable only with significant pressure
- Heavy fat deposits over lumbar area and base of tail
- Waist absent
- No abdominal tuck
- Obvious abdominal distension may be present

BCS 9

- Massive fat deposits over thorax, spine, and base of tail
- Waist and abdominal tuck absent
- Fat deposits on the neck and limbs
- Obvious abdominal distension

Body Condition Scoring System (Feline)[14]

Too Thin

BCS 1

- Ribs, spine, and pelvic bones easily visible on shorthaired cats
- Very narrow waist
- Small amount of muscle
- No palpable fat on the rib cage
- Severe abdominal tuck

BCS 2

- Ribs easily visible on shorthaired cats
- Very narrow waist
- Loss of muscle mass
- No palpable fat on the rib cage
- Very pronounced abdominal tuck

BCS 3

- Ribs visible on shorthaired cats
- Obvious waist
- Very small amount of abdominal fat
- Marked abdominal tuck

Continued

Body Condition Scoring System (Feline)[14]

BCS 4

- Ribs not visible but are easily palpable
- Obvious waist
- Minimal amount of abdominal fat

Ideal

BCS 5

- Well proportioned
- Ribs not visible but are easily palpable
- Obvious waist
- Small amount of abdominal fat
- Slight abdominal tuck

Overweight

BCS 6

- Ribs not visible but palpable
- Waist not clearly defined when seen from above
- Very slight abdominal tuck

BCS 7

- Ribs difficult to palpate under the fat
- Waist barely visible
- No abdominal tuck
- Rounding of abdomen with moderate abdominal pad

BCS 8

- Ribs not palpable under the fat
- Waist not visible
- Slight abdominal distension

BCS 9

- Ribs not palpable under a thick layer of fat
- Waist absent
- Obvious abdominal distension
- Extensive abdominal fat deposits

Resting Energy Requirements (RER) Calculation

$70 \times$ weight (kg) = calories/day
$30 \times$ weight (kg) + 70 = calories/day

Maintenance Energy Requirements

Canine Feeding Guide

Puppies	<4 months of age 3 × RER
	>4 months of age 2 × RER
Adult	1.6 × RER
Senior	1.4 × RER
Weight prevention	1.4 × RER
Weight loss	1.0 × RER
Gestation (last 21 days)	3.0 × RER
Lactation	4.0–8.0 × RER

Feline Feeding Guide

Kittens	2.5 × RER
Adult	1.2 × RER
Weight prevention	1.0 × RER
Weight loss	0.8 × RER
Breeding	1.6 × RER
Gestation (gradual increase)	2.0 × RER
Lactation	2.0–6.0 × RER

NUTRIENT GUIDELINES FOR WELLNESS[a,38]

Life Stage	Energy (kcal ME/g)	Protein	Fat	Fiber	Calcium	Phosphorus	Sodium
		Dry Matter					
Dog							
Growth/reproduction	3.5–5.0	22–35	10–25	5 max	0.7–1.7	0.6–1.3	0.35–0.6
Large-breed growth	3.0–4.0	22–35	8–12	10 max	0.7–1.2	0.6–1.1	0.3–0.6
Adult maintenance	3.5–4.5	15–30	10–20	5 max	0.5–1.0	0.4–0.9	0.2–0.4
Obesity prone	3.0–3.5	15–30	7–12	5–17	0.5–1.0	0.4–0.9	0.2–0.4
High energy	>4.5	22–34	26 min	5 max	0.5–1.0	0.4–0.9	0.2–0.5
Geriatric[b]	3.5–4.5	15–23	7–15	10 max	0.5–1.0	0.2–0.7	0.15–0.35

Continued

Life Stage	Energy (kcal ME/g)	Protein	Fat	Fiber	Calcium	Phosphorus	Sodium
		Dry Matter					
Cat							
Growth/reproduction	4.0–5.0	35–50	18–35	5 max	0.8–1.6	0.6–1.4	0.3–0.6
Adult maintenance	4.0–5.0	30–45	10–30	5 max	0.5–1.0	0.5–0.8	0.2–0.6
Obesity prone	3.3–3.8	30–45	8–17	5–15	0.5–1.0	0.5–0.9	0.2–0.6
Geriatric[b]	3.5–4.5	30–45	10–25	10 max	0.6–1.0	0.5–0.7	0.2–0.5

C, cup; *max*, maximum; *min*, minimum.

[a]Nutrients are expressed as % dry matter. Energy is expressed as kcal metabolizable energy (ME) per gram dry matter.

[b]Older animals require frequent body condition scoring. Feed intake adjustment may be required to maintain an ideal body condition, because some older individuals tend to be heavy and others tend to lose weight.

MUCUS MEMBRANES AND CAPILLARY REFILL TIME

MUCUS MEMBRANES

Photos	Mucus Membrane Color	Possible Interpretation	Possible Tests to Consider First
	Pink	Normal	Normal

Continued

Photos	Mucus Membrane Color	Possible Interpretation	Possible Tests to Consider First
	Gray or blue (cyanosis)[64]	Hypoxemia Oxygen immediately SPO_2>bell caps less than 75%	SPO_2 Radiographs

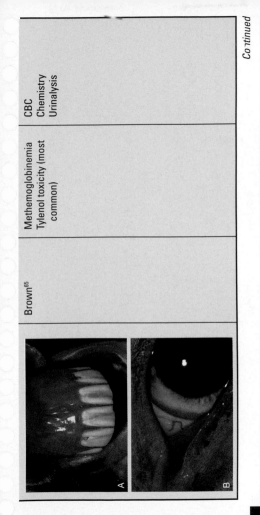

	Brown[65]	Methemoglobinemia Tylenol toxicity (most common)	CBC Chemistry Urinalysis

Photos	Mucus Membrane Color	Possible Interpretation	Possible Tests to Consider First
	Icterus[5]	Liver disease Hemolysis	Radiographs Ultrasound Blood smear CBC Chemistry Urinalysis
	White/pale[5]	Cardiogenic shock Anemia	CBC Blood smear Chemistry Urinalysis

	Brick red[5]	Heat stroke Septic shock Cyanide toxicity Carbon monoxide poisoning	Blood pressure CBC Chemistry Urinalysis
	Petechiae/ecchymosis	Coagulation problem DIC	CBC PT/PTT Chemistry Urinalysis

Capillary Refill Time (Sec)	Possible Interpretation
<1	Vasodilation Heat stroke Septic shock Systemic inflammatory response syndrome
1–2	Normal
>2.5	Vasoconstriction Hypovolemic shock Traumatic shock Cardiogenic shock

PAIN SCORES

Pain Score—Adapted From the Glasgow Scale

Select one option per question. Add the total points for all six sections.

Question 1—Is the Animal:

Quiet	0
Crying or whimpering	1
Groaning	2
Screaming	3

Question 2—Is the Animal:

Ignoring any wound or painful area	0
Looking at the wound or painful area	1

Pain Score—Adapted From the Glasgow Scale	
Licking wound or painful area	2
Rubbing wound or painful area	3
Chewing wound or painful area	4

Question 3—When the Animal Rises or Walks, Is It: (Do Not Complete if Fractures Suspected or Assistance in Locomotion Is Needed)

Normal	0
Lame	1
Slow or reluctant	2
Stiff	3
Refuses to move	4

Question 4: If the Animal Is Painful, How Do They React When Gentle Pressure Is Applied? (Do Not Complete if Fractures Are Suspect or Assistance in Locomotion Is Needed)

Do nothing	0
Look around	1
Flinch	2
Growl or guard area	3
Snap	4
Cry	5

Continued

Pain Score—Adapted From the Glasgow Scale	
Question 5: Overall the Animal Is:	
Happy and content or bouncy	0
Quiet	1
Indifferent or nonresponsive to surroundings	2
Nervous or anxious and fearful	3
Depressed or nonresponsive to stimulation	4
Question 6: Is the Animal:	
Comfortable	0
Unsettled	1
Restless	2
Hunched or tense	3
Rigid	4
Add points together from all six questions	Analgesic intervention is recommended at 6/24 or 5/20

ESTIMATING DEGREE OF DEHYDRATION

Evaluate Dehydration	
Degree of Dehydration	**Clinical Signs**
<5%	Not clinically detectable
5%–6%	Subtle loss of skin elasticity
6%–8%	Obvious delay in return of tented skin to normal position
	Slightly prolonged capillary refill time
	Eyes possibly sunken in orbits
	Possibly dry mucous membranes
10%–12%	Skin remains tented
	Very prolonged capillary refill time
	Eyes sunken in orbits
	Dry mucous membranes
	Possible signs of shock (tachycardia; cool extremities; rapid, weak pulse)
12%–15%	Obvious signs of shock
	Death imminent

PHYSICAL EXAM FINDINGS BY BODY SYSTEM

INTEGUMENT

Photos	Abnormality	Initial Tests to Consider
	Alopecia[72]: Hair loss	Skin scrape Trichogram DTM Impression smear Wood's lamp Fine needle aspirate Biopsy Excisional biopsy Thyroid testing CBC Chemistry

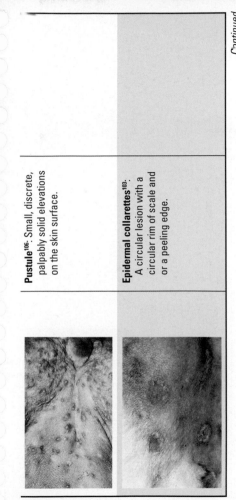

Pustule[106]: Small, discrete, palpably solid elevations on the skin surface.

Epidermal collarettes[103]: A circular lesion with a circular rim of scale and or a peeling edge.

Continued

Photos	Abnormality	Initial Tests to Consider
	Bulla⁶⁷: As above but more than 1 cm diameter.	
	Scale⁴¹: An accumulation of loose cornified fragments of the epidermis.	

Wheals: Circumscribed, raised lesion consisting of dermal edema.

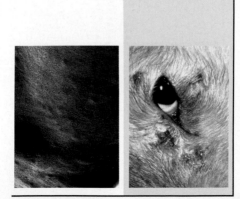

Vesicle[68A]**:** A small circumscribed elevation of the epidermis containing clear fluid less than 1 cm.

Continued

Photos	Abnormality	Initial Tests to Consider
	Papule[41]: Small, discrete, palpably solid elevations on the skin surface.	
	Macules[41]: Areas of discoloration of the skin, less than 1 cm in diameter. Typically erythematous, but they may be hyperpigmented.	

Continued

Crusts[33]: A dried exudate on the skin surface, either serum, blood, or pus or a combination.

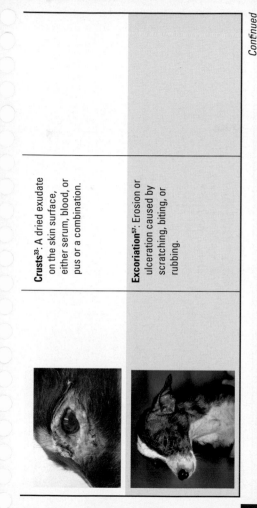

Excoriation[57]: Erosion or ulceration caused by scratching, biting, or rubbing.

Photos	Abnormality	Initial Tests to Consider
	Fissure[100,101]: Linear split through the epidermis into the underlying dermis.	
	Lichenification[106]: An accentuation of the skin markings giving an elephant skin–like appearance.	

Continued

Tumor: A large mass involving skin structures. The term is often used in relation to neoplasia but can technically be used in inflammatory disease.

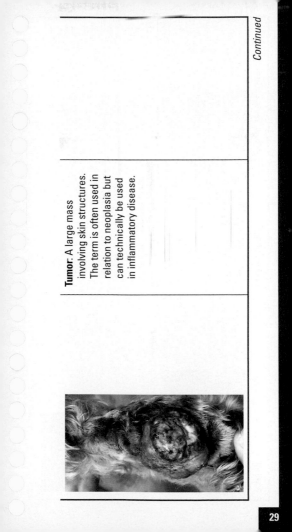

Photos	Abnormality	Initial Tests to Consider
	Cyst[66]. A cavity with an epithelial lining.	
	Nodule[68]. A solid elevation of the skin greater than 1 cm in diameter that usually extends into the deeper skin layers.	

Erosions/ulcers[57]: Superficial, whereas ulcers erode beneath the basement membrane, exposing the dermis.

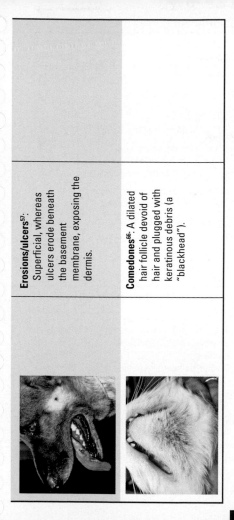

Comedones[56]: A dilated hair follicle devoid of hair and plugged with keratinous debris (a "blackhead").

RESPIRATORY

Respiratory	Tests to Consider
Rhythm	Radiographs
Upper airway auscultation	CBC
Nasal discharge	Chemistry
Rales: an abnormal rattling sound	SPO_2
Rhonchi: continuous gurgling or bubbling sounds typically heard during both inhalation and exhalation	
Crackles: brief, discontinuous, popping lung sounds that are high-pitched	
Dyspnea: difficult breathing	
Wheezing: a high-pitched, coarse whistling sound	

CARDIOVASCULAR

Cardiovascular-Heart murmur grade	Possible Tests to Consider
1/6—Can be heard in a quiet room only after several minutes of listening. **2/6**—Can be heard immediately but is very soft. **3/6**—Has low-to-moderate intensity. Patient is experiencing symptoms. **4/6**—Is loud but does not have a palpable thrill. **5/6**—Is loud with a palpable thrill. **6/6**—Can be heard with the stethoscope bell slightly off the thoracic wall.	Radiographs CBC Chemistry Urinalysis Echo-cardiogram

Character-Quality of the Murmur
- Plateau or regurgitant type (same sound for the duration of the murmur)
- Decrescendo, crescendo, crescendo–decrescendo, or ejection type (intensity changes throughout the duration of the murmur)
- Machinery (heard throughout systole and diastole)
- Decrescendo or blowing

Pulse Evaluation

Pulse Quality	Possible Interpretation
Weak	Cardiovascular collapse or shock
Bounding	Anemia, sepsis, or cardiac abnormalities

GASTROINTESTINAL

Gastrointestinal	Possible Tests to Consider
Diarrhea Vomiting Distention Abdominal wave Abdominal pain	Radiographs Fecal flotation Fecal smear CBC Chemistry Urinalysis Ultrasound Pancreatitis test Abdominocentesis

GENITOURINARY

Genitourinary	Possible Tests to Consider
Males: Testicular presence Penile discharge	Impression smear Radiographs Urinalysis Ultrasound CBC Chemistry Culture/sensitivity
Females: Evidence of pregnancy Lactation If intact, ask about the last heat cycle Vaginal discharge	

MUSCULOSKELETAL

Musculoskeletal	Possible Tests to Consider
Swelling Gait Guarding	Radiographs Lameness exam Ultrasound Tick screening CBC Chemistry

Lameness Scores

Grade 1	Sound at the walk, but weight shifting and mild lameness noted at trot
Grade 2	Mild weight-bearing lameness noted with the trained eye
Grade 3	Weight-bearing lameness, typically with distinct "head bob"
Grade 4	Significant weight-bearing lameness
Grade 5	Toe-touching lameness
Grade 6	Non–weight-bearing lameness

Patellar Luxation Grades

Grade 1	Patella can be manually luxated but returns to normal position.
Grade 2	Patella spontaneously luxates and returns to normal position. If patella is pushed out, it stays out.
Grade 3	Patella is out all the time but can be manually returned.
Grade 4	Patella is out continually and cannot be replaced.

Cranial Drawer

Cranial Drawer	Interpretation
Positive for tibial thrust[66]	Cranial cruciate ligament

Photos	Nervous System Abnormality	Possible Tests to Consider
	Horner's syndrome[69]: A persistently small pupil (miosis) A notable difference in pupil size between the two eyes (anisocoria) Little or delayed opening (dilation) of the affected pupil in dim light Drooping of the upper eyelid (ptosis) Elevation of the third eyelid Sunken appearance to the eye	Radiographs Tympanic membrane exam

	Radiographs CT/MRI
Proprioception[70]: Turn the paw over, so the top of the paw is sitting on the floor surface.	Radiographs CT/MRI
Motor: Pinch the webbing between the toes, so that the patient pulls the foot back.	

Continued

Photos	Nervous System Abnormality	Possible Tests to Consider
	Deep pain: Pinch the webbing between the toes, so that the patient feels the withdrawal. **Patellar reflex**[69]. Stimulate the patellar tendon with a plexor or hammer. A normal reaction is extension of the stifle. This is due to the femoral nerve, with nerve roots being usually between L4 and L6.	Radiographs CT/MRI

Triceps reflex[22]: Performed with the animal in lateral recumbency. The limb is supported under the radius. The triceps tendon is struck with a reflex hammer just proximal to the olecranon. Normal response is slight extension of the elbow branch of sciatic nerve.

Gastrocnemius reflex[22]: Flex and abduct the hock by holding the limb over the metatarsus; keep the hock flexed, which keeps the tendon tense. Tap the tendon. Evaluate L7–S1 spinal nerves and, peripherally, the tibial.

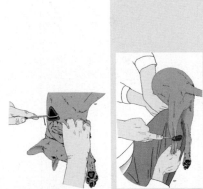

Continued

Photos	Nervous System Abnormality	Possible Tests to Consider

T12 dermatome
T13 dermatome
T11 dermatome
L1 dermatome
Iliac crest
C8–T1
Lateral thoracic nerve
Area of cutaneous trunci muscle
Costal arch | **Cutaneous trunci reflex**[69]. The sensory pathway from the skin enters the spinal cord and ascends bilaterally to the C8–T1 spinal cord segment, where it synapses with the lateral thoracic nerve, resulting in a contraction of the cutaneous trunci muscles bilaterally. | |

Cranial Nerves

- CN I: Olfactory nerve
- CN II: Optic nerve
- CN III: Oculomotor nerve
- CN IV: Trochlear nerve
- CN V: Trigeminal nerve
- CN VI: Abducens nerve
- CN VII: Facial nerve
- CN VIII: Vestibulocochlear nerve
- CN IX: Glossopharyngeal nerve
- CN X: Vagus nerve
- CN XI: Accessory nerve
- CN XII: Hypoglossal nerve

Cranial Nerves Tests	
Menace response	A: CN II (retina); E: CN VI, CN VII; in addition, the thalamus, cerebrum, and cerebellum are involved in the response and its pathway
Palpebral reflex	A: CN V; E: CN VII
Vibrissae (and maxilla) response	A: CN V (maxillary branch); E: CN VII; this response also involves the cerebrum
Mandibular touch	A: CN V (mandibular branch); E: CN VII
Auricular reflex	A: CN VII; E: CN VII

Continued

Cranial Nerves Tests	
Corneal reflex: The cornea is touched lightly with a moist cotton tip applicator; the eye should retract.	A: CN V (ophthalmic branch); E: CN VI
Pupillary light reflex (PLR): Performed in a dark room to assess anisocoria (unequal pupil size). Indirect PLR is usually not as strong as direct PLR.	A: CN II; E: CN III

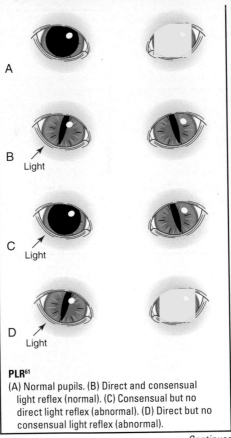

A

B
Light

C
Light

D
Light

PLR[61]
(A) Normal pupils. (B) Direct and consensual light reflex (normal). (C) Consensual but no direct light reflex (abnormal). (D) Direct but no consensual light reflex (abnormal).

Continued

Cranial Nerves Tests	
Oculocephalic reflex normal physiologic nystagmus: Palpation of the head for symmetry. Assess for asymmetry, muscle atrophy, and droopy lips.	A: CN VIII; E: CN III, IV, and VI Muscles of mastication are innervated by CN V (mandibular motor branch); muscles of facial expression are innervated by CN VII
Gag reflex	A: CN IX; E: CN X
Palpation of the neck to assess muscle atrophy	E: CN XI (difficult to assess)
Tongue movement and symmetry	E: CN XII

Photos	Ocular Abnormality	Tests to Consider
	Abrasions, ulcers, discharge.	Intraocular pressure Fluorescein stain Schirmer tear test Orbital exam

Continued

Photos	Ocular Abnormality	Tests to Consider
	Lenticular sclerosis: Bluish discoloration on the pupil: *when using an ophthalmoscope, you can see through the lens to the retina. You are not able to do this with a cataract.*	Normal aging process

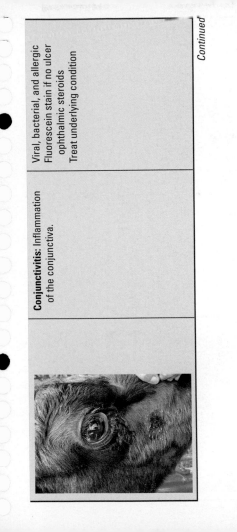

	Conjunctivitis: Inflammation of the conjunctiva.	Viral, bacterial, and allergic Fluorescein stain if no ulcer ophthalmic steroids Treat underlying condition

Continued

Photos	Ocular Abnormality	Tests to Consider
	Hyphema: Blood in the anterior chamber.	*Look for systemic disease or coagulopathy*
	Hypopyon: Creamy white to yellow opacity noted in the ventral anterior chamber.	*Look for systemic disease*

	Lens luxation: Portion of pupil no longer containing the lens.	**Acute** anterior lens luxation is considered an emergency. Posterior, topical miotic treatment can restrict lens movement. Referral
	Cataracts[33]: Opaque pupillary opening, progressive vision loss; inherited or secondary to diabetes and other diseases.	Check IOP Topical mydriatics and antiinflammatories Surgery

Continued

Photos	Ocular Abnormality	Tests to Consider
	Entropion inversion of part or the entire eyelid margin toward the eye.[33]	Surgery
	Ectropion eversion of part or the entire eyelid.	Surgery

Retinal degeneration[33]. Visual disturbances to blindness: inherited or idiopathic (SARD).		Retinal exam: no treatment
Proptosis[33]. Globe of the eyelid protruding from the orbit.		Surgery

Continued

Photos	Ocular Abnormality	Tests to Consider
	Distichiasis/ectopic cilia[33]: Epiphora, blepharospasm, mild conjunctivitis, and keratitis.	Check for entropion surgery
	Ruptured cornea[33]: Perforation of the cornea.	Enucleation

Otic	Tests to Consider
Pain, odor, ulcers, and discharge	Ear cytology Ear mite exam Culture/sensitivity Gram stain

Dental Score	Photos	Tests to Consider
Grade 1		Radiographs
Grade 2		CBC

			Chemistry
Grade 3			
Grade 4			Comprehensive Oral Health Assessment and Treatment

LYMPHATICS

Lymphatics	Tests to Consider
If all are swollen, think systemic disease or lymphoma	Lymph node aspirate Biopsy CBC Chemistry Urinalysis Radiographs

Location of Palpable Lymph Nodes[57]

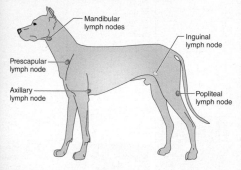

Mandibular lymph nodes

Inguinal lymph node

Prescapular lymph node

Axillary lymph node

Popliteal lymph node

RECTAL EXAM

Rectal Exam	Tests to Consider
Prostate Anal glands Masses	Radiographs CBC Chemistry Urinalysis

HEMATOLOGY, SEROLOGY, AND URINALYSIS

ANTICOAGULANTS[51]

Order of Draw	Cap Color		Additive	Primary Use
First	Light blue		Sodium citrate	Coagulation studies
	Red		Glass: no additive Plastic: silicon-coated	Serum for blood chemistry
	Red/gray, gold, or red/black "tiger-top"		Gel separator and clot activator	
	Green or tan		Heparin	Plasma for blood chemistry
	Lavender, royal blue, or tan		EDTA	Hematology
Last	Gray		Potassium oxalate or sodium fluoride	Coagulation testing Glucose testing

HEMATOLOGY REFERENCE RANGE VALUES[21]

Test	Adult Canine	Adult Feline	Units	Changes	Possible Interpretations
Red blood cell (total)	5.32–7.75	6.68–11.8	×10^6 cells/µL	Elevated	Dehydration Splenic contraction Polycythemia
				Decreased (anemia)	Regenerative anemia Nonregenerative anemia Hemolytic anemia Idiopathic aplastic anemia Red cell aplasia Myeloproliferative disease Myelophthisis Hypersplenism Lead poisoning Leukemia

Test	Adult Canine	Adult Feline	Units	Changes	Possible Interpretations
Hemoglobin (Hgb)	13.5–19.5	11.0–15.8	g/dL		Usually proportional to hematocrit, except where hemoglobin synthesis defects stimulate polycythemia
Hematocrit (Hct)	39.4–56.2	33.6–50.2	%	Elevated	Dehydration (total protein will also be increased) Polycythemia Splenic contracture
				Decreased	Anemias: see RBC

| Mean corpuscular volume | 65.7–75.7 | 42.6–55.5 | fL | Increased (macrocytosis)—Will appear as reticulocytes with NMB stain | Artifact (extended time in EDTA) Regenerative anemia FELV FIV Greyhounds and Poodles Bone marrow disease Vitamin B_{12} deficiency |
| $MCV = \dfrac{Hct \times 10}{RBC\ count}$ | | | | Decreased (microcytosis) | Artifact Iron deficiency Portosystemic shunt Polycythemia Breeds (Akita, Shar-pei, and Shiba Inu) |

Continued

Test	Adult Canine	Adult Feline	Units	Changes	Possible Interpretations
Mean corpuscular hemoglobin (MCH)	22.57–27.0	13.4–18.6	pg		Utilize MCHC
Mean corpuscular hemoglobin concentration (MCHC) $$MCHC = \frac{Hb\ (g/dL) \times 100}{Hct}$$	34.3–36.0	31.3–33.5	g/dL	Increased (hyperchromic) Decreased (hypochromic)	Lipemia Hemolysis RBC shape changes (Heinz bodies and spherocytes) Regeneration Iron deficiency

| Platelet count | 194–419 | 198–405 | $\times 10^3$ cells/μL | Increased (thrombocytosis) | Excited
Chronic bleeding
Iron deficiency
Inflammation
Neoplasia
Cushing's
Essential thrombocytosis
Rebound thrombocytosis
Polycythemia vera |
| | | | | Decreased (thrombocytopenia)
Less than 100,000/μL
Spontaneous bleeding will occur at less than 25,000/μL | FELV
FIV
Ehrlichia
Immune-mediated thrombocytopenia
Hypersplenism
Hemorrhage
DIC
King Charles Spaniels
Greyhounds |

Continued

Test	Adult Canine	Adult Feline	Units	Changes	Possible Interpretations
Platelet estimate methods[51]					
1. Number of platelets averaged over 10 fields on peripheral blood smear × 15,000–20,000					
2. Total number of platelets per 100 RBCs multiplied by the RBC count divided by 1000 = platelet estimate × 10⁹/L					
$$\frac{\text{Thrombocytes}}{100 \text{ leukocytes}} \times \frac{\text{WBC count}}{\mu L} = \frac{\text{thrombocytes}}{\mu L}$$					
Mean platelet volume	8.8–14.3	11.3–21.3	fL	Increased	Bone marrow disease (confirm with blood smear)

| White blood cell (total) | 4.36–14.8 | 4.79–12.52 | ×10³ cells/μL | Elevated (leukocytosis) | Infection
Physiologic
Stress
Glucocorticoids
Immune-mediated disease
Neoplasia
Tissue trauma
Tissue necrosis
Leukemia
Hemorrhagic anemia
Hemolytic anemia |
| | | | | Decreased (leukopenia) | Decreased production
Increased consumption |

Continued

Test	Adult Canine	Adult Feline	Units	Changes	Possible Interpretations
Segmented neutrophils (segs)	3.4–9.8	1.6–15.6	×10³ cells/ μL	Increased (neutrophilia)	Stress Infection Immune-mediated disease Neoplasia Tissue trauma Tissue necrosis Cushing's Steroids Uremia Diabetic ketoacidosis Regenerative anemia Leukemia

	Decreased (neutropenia)			
	Myeloproliferative disease			
	Lymphoproliferative diseases			
	Neoplasia			
	Myelofibrosis			
	Drug induced			
	Overwhelming infection (parvovirus, pyometra, and sepsis)			
	Addison's			
	Ehrlichiosis			
	FIV			
	FELV			
	Hypersplenism			
	Immune mediated			

Continued

Test	Adult Canine	Adult Feline	Units	Changes	Possible Interpretations
Lymphocytes (lymphs)	0.8–3.5	1.0–7.4	$\times 10^3$ cells/μL	Increased (lymphocytosis)	Physiologic Epinephrine induced Postvaccination leukemia Chronic infections Immune mediated Inflammatory bowel disease Cholangiohepatitis Ehrlichiosis Chagas disease Babesiosis Leishmaniasis Addison's

Monocytes (mono)	0.2–1.1	0–0.7	×10³ cells/µL	Decreased (lymphopenia) Stress Cushing's Chemotherapy FELV FIV Chylothorax Lymphangiectasia FIP Parvovirus Canine distemper Canine infectious hepatitis	Increased monocytosis Infections Stress Steroids Immune mediated Trauma with severe crushing Hemorrhage Neoplasia

Continued

Test	Adult Canine	Adult Feline	Units	Changes	Possible Interpretations
Eosinophils (eos)	0–1.9	0.1–2.3	×10³ cells/µL	Elevated (eosinophilia)	Parasites Allergies Eosinophilic granuloma complex Feline asthma Eosinophilic gastroenteritis Hypereosinophilic syndrome Supportive processes Toxoplasmosis Neoplasia Addison's Pregnancy
				Decreased (eosinopenia)	Stress Cushing's Steroid therapy

| Basophils (basos) | 0 | 0 | ×10³ cells/μL | Elevated (basophilia) | Heartworm disease Allergies GI tract disease Respiratory tract disease Neoplasia Hyperlipoproteinemia |

DIC, Disseminated intravascular coagulation; *FELV*, feline leukemia virus; *FIV*, feline immunodeficiency virus; *MMB*, new methylene blue.

HEMOSTASIS REFERENCE RANGE VALUES[21]

Tests	Canine	Feline	Change	Possible Interpretation	Three of Below Indicates DIC
Prothrombin time (PT)	5.1–7.9 sec	8.4–10.8 sec	Prolonged	Deficiencies of II, VII, and X Vitamin K antagonists (rodenticide poisoning) Bile insufficiency Liver failure	◆
			Decreased	Unremarkable	

Continued

Tests	Canine	Feline	Change	Possible Interpretation	Three of Below Indicates DIC
Activated partial thromboplastin time (APTT)	8.6–12.9 sec	13.7–30.2 sec	Prolonged	Deficiencies of VIII, IX, XI, XII, and fibrinogen Von Willebrand disease Vitamin K antagonists (rodenticide poisoning) Coumarin poisoning Bile insufficiency Liver failure Hemophilia A Hemophilia B	◆
			Decreased	Unremarkable	
Fibrin degradation products	<10 μg/mL	<10 μg/mL	Increased	Clot-dissolving activity	◆
			Decreased	Unremarkable	

	100–245 mg/dL	110–370 mg/dL	Increased Decreased		Inflammation Unremarkable	◆
Fibrinogen	100–245 mg/dL	110–370 mg/dL	Increased Decreased		Inflammation Unremarkable	◆
Activated clotting time	60–110 sec	50–75 sec	Prolonged		Screening test for II, V, VIII, IX, X, XI, and XII Severe thrombocytopenia Decreased fibrinogen	
D-Dimer (assays for breakdown of fibrin clots)			Decreased Negative	Decreased	Unremarkable Negative reliable rules out DIC	◆
Platelet count			Decreased		See above	◆

HEMATOLOGY MORPHOLOGY

Photos	Name	Possible Interpretations	
	Normal RBC[83] (normocytic)—biconcave disks in mammals	Normal	

Continued

Elliptocyte[76]	Normal for llama, avian, reptiles, and fish	
Anisocytosis[51]—variation in size of RBCs	Splenic disorders Liver disorders Regenerative anemia	

Photos	Name	Possible Interpretations
	Acanthocyte[25,51,54,63] irregular projections from RBC surface	Liver disease Splenic disease Fragmentation disorders
	Codocyte[25,51,54,63] Bull's eye appearance, AKA target cell	Liver disease Iron-deficiency anemia Splenic disease

	Drepanocyte[82] (sickle cell)	Nonpathogenic in goats
	Echinocyte[25,51,54,63] scalloped border of RBC surface	Artifact Uremia Pyruvate kinase deficiency

Photos	Name	Possible Interpretations
	Keratocyte[76]	Fragmentation hemolysis Iron deficiency anemia
	Schistocyte[54]—fragmented RBC	DIC Vasculitis Cancer Fragmentation hemolysis Iron deficiency anemia

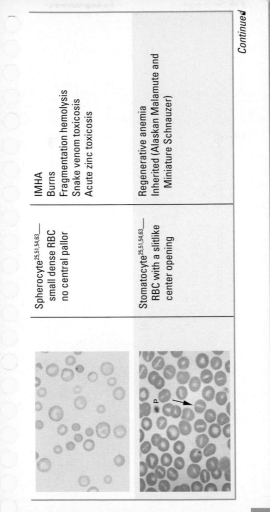

| | Spherocyte[25,51,54,63] small dense RBC no central pallor | IMHA
Burns
Fragmentation hemolysis
Snake venom toxicosis
Acute zinc toxicosis |
| | Stomatocyte[25,51,54,63] RBC with a slitlike center opening | Regenerative anemia
Inherited (Alaskan Malamute and Miniature Schnauzer) |

Continued

Photos	Name	Possible Interpretations
	Basophilic stippling[25]—bluish granular bodies on the surface of the RBC	Regenerative anemia in ruminants Lead poisoning

| | Heinz bodies[25]—round structures within the RBC | Small numbers normal in cats
Onion toxicity
Tylenol toxicity |
| | Nucleated RBC[28,51] | Regenerative anemia
Lead poisoning
Extramedullary hematopoiesis
Bone marrow disease |

Continued

Photos	Name	Possible Interpretations
	Reticulocytes[37]	Reticulocyte count[37] $$\frac{\text{\# of reticulocytes}}{1000 \text{ RBCs}} \times 100 = \% \text{ reticulocytes}$$ Corrected reticulocyte perunit = $$\frac{\% \text{ reticulocytes} \times \text{patient's PCV}}{45(\text{dog}) \text{ or } 37(\text{cat})}$$
	Mycoplasma[28,51]-on the periphery of RBC	

Note: *IMHA*, Immune-mediated hemolytic anemia.

82

WBC MORPHOLOGY

Photos	Name	Possible Interpretations
	Normal Neutrophils[28]	
	Normal Lymphocytes[76]	

Continued

Photos	Name	Possible Interpretations
	Normal Monocytes[28]	
	Normal Eosinophils[76]	

Normal
Basophils[54]

Band[18,26,31,51] — immature WBC, usually neutrophils. Nonsegmented nucleus, nuclear sides are usually parallel

Corrected WBC count[51]

$$\text{Corrected WBC count} = \text{observed WBC count} \times \frac{\%\ \text{NRBCs}}{100\ \text{WBCs}}$$

Continued

Photos	Name	Possible Interpretations
	Hypersegmented neutrophil[18,26,31,51]___ neutrophil nucleus with more than six lobes	Chronic infection Pernicious anemia Steroid therapy
	Karyorrhexis/ karyolysis/ pyknosis[18,26,31,51]___ describes a nucleus that is condensed, lysed, or damaged	Inappropriate anticoagulants

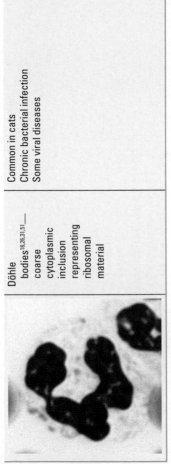

Döhle bodies[18,26,31,51] — coarse cytoplasmic inclusion representing ribosomal material

Common in cats
Chronic bacterial infection
Some viral diseases

Continued

Photos	Name	Possible Interpretations
	Vacuolization[18,26,31,51]___ one of several toxic changes seen in both lymphocytes and neutrophils Normal in monocytes	Artifact Septicemia

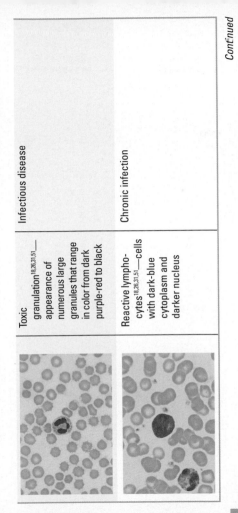	Toxic granulation[18,26,31,51]—appearance of numerous large granules that range in color from dark purple-red to black	Infectious disease
	Reactive lymphocytes[18,26,31,51]—cells with dark-blue cytoplasm and darker nucleus	Chronic infection

Continued

Photos	Name	Possible Interpretations
	Atypical lymphocytes[18,26,31,51]___ a variety of changes in lymphocytes including eosinophilic cytoplasm and changes in nuclear texture	
	Basket cell, nuclear streaming, smudge cells[18,26,31,51]___ common term used to describe and degenerative WBC that have ruptured	Artifact Leukemia

NORMAL CHEMISTRY[21]

Test	Adult Canine	Adult Feline	Units	Change	Possible Interpretations
Glucose	73–116	63–150	mg/dL	Increased (hyperglycemia)	Stress Diabetes mellitus Cushing's Pancreatitis Drug induced Iatrogenic Postprandial Acromegaly Diestrus Pheochromocytoma Neoplasia Renal insufficiency Head trauma

Continued

Test	Adult Canine	Adult Feline	Units	Change	Possible Interpretations
				Decreased (hypoglycemia)	Prolonged sample storage Hepatic insufficiency Sepsis Iatrogenic Toxicity Neoplasia Leukemia Addison's Hypopituitarism Idiopathic Neonatal Renal failure Glycogen storage disease Severe polycythemia Starvation

Blood urea nitrogen (BUN)	8–27	15–35	mg/dL	Increased	Kidney failure
					Dehydration
					Shock
					Diet
					GI bleeding
					Toxins
					Rhabdomyolysis
				Decreased	Liver failure
					Diet
					Polydipsia/polyuria
					GI flora changes in large animals
					Cushing's
					Overzealous fluid therapy
					Steroid use
					Diabetes insipidus
					Neonates

Continued

Test	Adult Canine	Adult Feline	Units	Change	Possible Interpretations
Creatinine (Cr)	0.5–1.6	0.5–2.3	mg/dL	Increased	Renal disease Rhabdomyolysis Greyhounds Draft Horses Postprandial ferrets
				Decreased	Decreased muscle Sepsis Hyperbilirubinemia
Azotemia	Elevation of BUN and CRE				Renal disease Urinary obstruction Dehydration Cushing's Heart failure Shock

| Phosphorus (P) | 2.0–6.7 | 2.7–7.6 | mg/dL | Increased | Delayed serum separation
Growing animals
Renal failure
Postrenal obstruction
Primary hypoparathyroidism
Nutritional secondary hyperparathyroidism
Hyperthyroidism
Acromegaly
Hemolysis
Toxicity
Hypoparathyroidism
Dietary excess |

Continued

Test	Adult Canine	Adult Feline	Units	Change	Possible Interpretations
				Decreased	Metabolic acidosis Iatrogenic Osteolysis Neoplasia Rhabdomyolysis Primary hyperparathyroidism Nutritional secondary hyperparathyroidism Renal tubular acidosis Vomiting Diarrhea Neoplasia Insulin therapy Diabetic ketoacidosis Fanconi syndrome

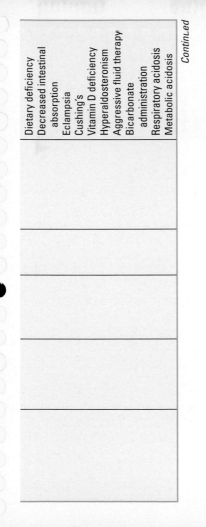

Dietary deficiency				
Decreased intestinal absorption				
Eclampsia				
Cushing's				
Vitamin D deficiency				
Hyperaldosteronism				
Aggressive fluid therapy				
Bicarbonate administration				
Respiratory acidosis				
Metabolic acidosis				

Continued

Test	Adult Canine	Adult Feline	Units	Change	Possible Interpretations
Calcium (Ca)	9.2–11.6	7.5–11.5	mg/dL	Increased	Primary hyperparathyroidism Renal failure Addison's Neoplasia Toxicity Dehydration Systemic mycosis FIP Osteomyelitis HOD Iatrogenic Serum lipemia Postprandial Idiopathic (cats) Lab error

	Decreased
	Renal failure
	Acute pancreatitis
	Intestinal malabsorption
	Primary hypoparathyroidism
	Eclampsia
	Ethylene glycol toxicity
	Hypoproteinemia
	Hypoalbuminemia
	Hypomagnesemia
	Nutritional secondary hyperparathyroidism
	Neoplasia
	Phosphate containing enemas
	Anticonvulsant medications

Continued

Test	Adult Canine	Adult Feline	Units	Change	Possible Interpretations
Total protein (TP)	5.5–7.2	5.4–8.9	g/dL	Increased	Dehydration Chronic inflammation Neoplasia Hemolysis Lipemia
					Hypovitaminosis D Rhabdomyolysis Sodium bicarbonate administration Lab error

| Albumin (Alb) | 2.8–4.0 | 3.0–4.2 | g/dL | Decreased | Hemorrhage
Hypoalbuminemia
Liver failure
External plasma loss
GI fluid loss
Malassimilation
Starvation
Overhydration
Glomerular loss
Neoplasia |
| | | | | Increased | Dehydration
Hemolysis
Lipemia
Laboratory error |

Continued

Test	Adult Canine	Adult Feline	Units	Change	Possible Interpretations
				Decreased	Protein-losing nephropathy Gastroenteropathy Liver failure Malnutrition Parasites Vasculitis Burns Abrasions Degloving Neonates External blood loss Chronic effusions Hyperglobulinemia Multiple myeloma

Globulin (Glob)	2.0–4.1	2.8–5.3	g/dL	Increased	Dehydration Infection Immune mediated Neoplasia
				Decreased	Unremarkable
Cholesterol (Ch)	138–317	42–265	mg/dL	Increased	Postprandial Primary hyperlipidemia Endocrine disease Cholestasis Dietary Nephrotic syndrome Protein-losing nephropathy Idiopathic in Doberman Pinscher and Rottweiler

Continued

Test	Adult Canine	Adult Feline	Units	Change	Possible Interpretations
				Decreased	Liver failure Malabsorption Maldigestion Protein-losing enteropathy Portosystemic shunt Lymphangiectasia Starvation Addison's Neoplasia
Bilirubin (total)	0–0.2	0.1–0.5	mg/dL	Increased	Liver disease Gallbladder disease Hemolytic anemia Pancreatitis Neoplasia Nodular hyperplasia Feline hepatic lipidosis Duodenal perforation
				Decreased	Unremarkable

Alkaline phosphatase (SAP or ALP or AP)	15–146	0–96	IU/L	Increased	Liver disease Bone growth and disease Gallbladder Endocrine disorders Steroid use Anticonvulsant use
				Decreased	Unremarkable
Alanine aminotrans-ferase (ALT) formally SGPT	16–73	5–134	IU/L	Increased	Liver disease
				Decreased	End-stage liver disease
					Unremarkable
Aspartate aminotrans-ferase (AST) formerly SGOT				Increased	Liver or muscle injury in large animals Hyperthyroidism
				Decreased	Unremarkable

Continued

Test	Adult Canine	Adult Feline	Units	Change	Possible Interpretations
Gamma glutamyl-transferase (GGT)	3–8	0–10	IU/L	Increased	Mirrors ALP Cats with hepatic lipidosis tend to have normal to mildly elevated GGT but greatly elevated ALP
				Decreased	Lipemic samples Hemolysis Laboratory error
Creatine kinase (CK; formerly CPK)	48–380	72–481	IU/L	Increased	Muscle damage Pyrexia Hypothermia Cardiomyopathy DIC
				Decreased	Unremarkable

Sodium (Na)	147–154	147–165	IU/L	Increased	Dehydration Renal failure Vomiting/diarrhea Panting Fever Pancreatitis Peritonitis Burns Hyperaldosteronism Increased salt intake
				Decrease	Addison's Vomiting/diarrhea Liver disease Hookworms Renal failure Chronic effusions

Continued

Test	Adult Canine	Adult Feline	Units	Change	Possible Interpretations
					Diuretics Hypotonic fluids Diabetes mellitus Burns Excess antidiuretic hormone Diet Antidiuretic drugs Psychogenic polydipsia Hyperlipidemia Hyperproteinemia

Potassium (K)	3.9–5.2	3.3–5.7	mEq/L	Elevated
				Renal failure
				Urinary obstruction
				Ruptured bladder
				Addison's
				Acidosis
				GI disease
				Massive muscle trauma
				Dehydration
				Diuretics
				Thrombocytosis
				Severe leukocytosis
				Hemolysis
				Hyperkalemic periodic paralysis

Continued

Test	Adult Canine	Adult Feline	Units	Change	Possible Interpretations
				Decreased	Alkalosis
					Diet
					Bicarbonate administration
					Potassium-free fluids
					Drugs
					Vomiting/diarrhea
					Cushing's
					Hyperaldosteronism
					Insulin therapy
					Diuresis
					Hypokalemic periodic paralysis
					Renal failure
					Total parenteral nutrition

A:G ratio	0.6–2.0		
Na:K ratio	27.4–38.4	30–43	—	Suggestive of Addison's
Chloride (Cl)	104–117	113–122	—	
Bicarbonate (venous)	20–29	22–24	mEq/L	
Anion gap	16.3–28.6	15–32	mEq/L	Elevated Lactic acidosis Uremia Ketoacidosis Ethylene glycol toxicity Decreased Hypalbuminemia IgG multiple myeloma

Continued

Test	Adult Canine	Adult Feline	Units	Change	Possible Interpretations
Anion gap calculation	[Na+K]−[Cl−HCO3−] = Anion gap				
Osmolality (calculated)	292–310	290–320		Greater than 280 mOsm/kg	Suggests central DI Nephrogenic DI Psychogenic polydipsia Primary polyuria
				Less than 280 mOsm/kg	Suggests psychogenic polydipsia Diabetic ketoacidosis Azotemia Hypernatremia Hyperglycemia Ethylene glycol toxicity

	347–1104	489–2100	mOsm/kg		
Amylase				Increased	May not correlate with severity of disease. Not very sensitive or specific especially in cats. Pancreatic disease Renal disease
				Decreased	Unremarkable
Lipase	22–216	0–222	IU/L	Increased	Not very sensitive or specific for pancreatic disease Pancreatic disease Enteritis Renal disease Hepatic disease Steroids

Continued

Test	Adult Canine	Adult Feline	Units	Change	Possible Interpretations
Triglyceride (TG)	19–133	24–206	mg/dL	Increased	Postprandial Familial triglyceridemia Hyperchylomicronemia Lipoprotein lipase deficiency (cats) Endocrine disease Nephrotic syndrome Pancreatitis Cholestasis Steroids
				Decreased	Not clearly associated with any disease

	Preprandial 0–0.5 Postprandial 5.0–25.0	Preprandial 0–0.5 Postprandial 1–20.0	µmol/L		
Bile acids (Fasting is best) Cannot be icteric				Increased	Liver disease Portosystemic shunt Cholestasis
				Decreased	Delayed gastric emptying Malabsorption Rapid intestinal transport
Thyroxine: total serum T_4				Increased	Cats—hyperthyroidism
					Euthyroid
				Decreased	Hypothyroidism
Free T_4 by equilibrium dialysis				Increased	Hyperthyroidism
				Decreased	Hypothyroidism—Note: A free T4 by ED is required to confirm Hypothyroidism in Dogs
Canine thyroid-stimulating hormone				Normal	Rules out hypothyroidism
				Decreased	Supports hypothyroidism

URINALYSIS GROSS EXAM, SPECIFIC GRAVITY, AND STICK EVALUATION[21]

Test	Normal Canine	Normal Feline	Abnormalities	Possible Interpretations
Daily urine output (mL/kg)	20–40	20–40	Increased (polyuria)	Renal insufficiency Renal failure Diabetes mellitus Cushing's disease UTI Urolith Cancer Anatomic problem Neurological problem Pyometra Hypoadrenocorticism Hypocalcemia Addison's disease

	Polakiuria (frequent abnormal urination)			
	Pyelonephritis			
	Hypokalemia			
	Iatrogenic			
	Hyperthyroidism			
	Hepatic insufficiency			
	Postobstructive			
	Diabetes insipidus			
	Psychogenic drinking			
	Renal glucosuria			
	Uroliths			
	UTI			
	Improper litter box management			

Continued

Test	Normal Canine	Normal Feline	Abnormalities	Possible Interpretations
			Decreased (oliguria) No production (anuria)	Obstruction Dehydration Hypovolemia Acute renal failure (toxic, infectious, ischemia, immune mediated) Cancer Systemic disease with renal manifestations (infections, pancreatitis, sepsis, multiple organ failure, heart failure, SLE, hepatorenal disease)

	1.020–1.050	1.025–1.060	Increased	Risk for FLUTD
Specific gravity (SpGr)			Isosthenuria (1.008–1.012)	Renal failure
				PU/PD (see above)
			Hyposthenuria (less than 1.008)	Diabetes insipidus
Color	Pale-to-dark yellow	Pale-to-dark yellow	Colorless	Dilute urine with low SG
			Deep amber	Highly concentrated urine (high SG)
			White	Associated with presence of leukocytes
			Red to red/brown	Usually indicates presence of RBCs, hemoglobin, or myoglobinuria
			Dark brown or black	Methemoglobinuria

Continued

Test	Normal Canine	Normal Feline	Abnormalities	Possible Interpretations
Turbidity	Clear	Clear	Cloudy	Usually indicates presence of cells (e.g., WBCs, mucus, crystals, epithelial cells, and bacteria)
			Milky	Usually indicates presence of fatty material
pH	5.0–7.5	5.0–7.5	Less than 5.0	Meat-based diet Iatrogenic Metabolic acidosis Respiratory acidosis Protein catabolic states Severe vomiting with chloride depletion

Protein	Negative to +1 (0–30 mg/dL)	Negative to +1	Greater than +1	Interpret in light of specific gravity Glomerular disease Inflammatory disease
			Greater than 7.5	Vegetable-based diet Iatrogenic UTI Postparangial Metabolic alkalosis Respiratory alkalosis Renal tubular acidosis
Glucose	Negative	Negative	Positive	Diabetes mellitus Stress Iatrogenic Pheochromocytoma Acute renal failure Fanconi syndrome Primary renal glucosuria

Continued

Test	Normal Canine	Normal Feline	Abnormalities	Possible Interpretations
Ketones	Negative	Negative	Positive	Diabetic ketoacidosis Starvation Glycogen storage disease Low-carbohydrate diet Persistent fever Persistent hypoglycemia
Bilirubin	Negative to trace	Negative	Positive	Hemolysis Liver disease Extrahepatic obstruction Fever Starvation
Blood (hematuria)	Negative	Negative	Positive	In heat Inflammation Urolithiasis Obstruction Trauma

Urine protein: creatinine	<0.3	<0.6	Increased	Cancer Bleeding disorders Heat stroke Renal infarct Granulomatous urethritis FLUTD Parasitism Drug induced Renal pelvic hematoma Vascular malformation Idiopathic Renal telangiectasia (Welsh Corgi) Rental hematuria (Weimaraners) Pseudohematuria More accurate than the dipstick protein estimation to assess proteinuria

Note: Other parameters that can be tested using urinary stick analysis are not listed in this table because those parameters are traditionally not accurate and should not be trusted.

FLUTD, Feline lower urinary tract disease; *PU/PD*, polyuria/polydipsia; *SG*, specific gravity; *SLE*, systemic lupus erythematosus; *UTI*, urinary tract infection.

URINARY CELLULAR SEDIMENT EXAMINATION

LOWER THE LIGHT SOURCE TO INCREASE CONTRAST! USE OF SEDI-STAIN MAY IMPROVE VISUALIZATION

Photos	Name	Cat and Dog Normal	Possible Interpretation
	RBC[54,62]	<5 RBCs/hpf	See hematuria above

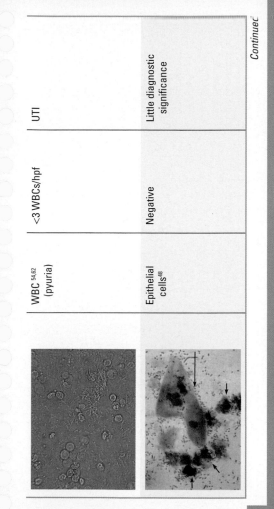

WBC [54,62] (pyuria)	<3 WBCs/hpf	UTI
Epithelial cells [48]	Negative	Little diagnostic significance

Continued

Photos	Name	Cat and Dog Normal	Possible Interpretation
	Transitional cells[48]	Negative	Little diagnostic significance, but can mean infection, neoplasia, or irritation
	Bacteria[90]	Negative	UTI

Pearsonema spp. Ovum[47]	Negative	Parasite infection

URINALYSIS CAST SEDIMENT EXAMINATION—NO CASTS SHOULD BE PRESENT

Photos	Name	Possible Interpretation
	Hyaline Cast[12]	Glomerulonephritis Amyloidosis Small numbers can be seen with fever and exercise

| Granular Cast[49] | Ischemic or nephrotoxic renal tubular injury | |
| WBC Casts[105] | Pyelonephritis | |

Photos	Name	Possible Interpretation
	Red Cell Casts[16,49]	Intrarenal hemorrhage (rare)
	Renal Epithelial Casts[16,49]	Acute tubular necrosis Pyelonephritis

Fatty Casts[105]	Nephrotic syndrome Diabetes mellitus	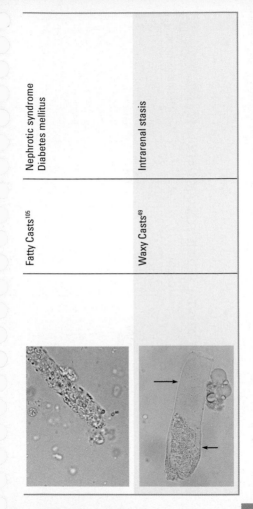
Waxy Casts[49]	Intrarenal stasis	

URINE CRYSTAL SEDIMENT EXAMINATION

Photos	Crystal	pH	Possible Interpretation
	Ammonium biurate[84]	Any slightly acidic, neutral, alkaline	Can be normal in Dalmatians, English Bulldogs, and Black Russian Terriers Congenital or acquired portal vascular anomalies Chemotherapy

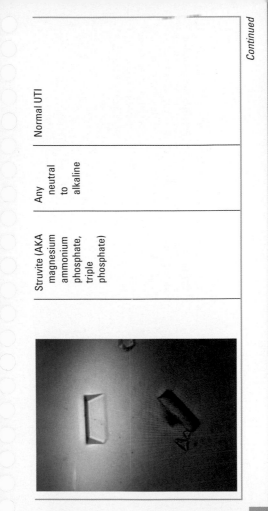

	Struvite (AKA magnesium ammonium phosphate, triple phosphate)	Any neutral to alkaline	Normal UTI

Continued

Photos	Crystal	pH	Possible Interpretation
	Amorphous urates[49]	Acidic, neutral	These crystals occur in Dalmatians on allopurinol therapy for urate urolithiasis. Easily confused with bacteria

Bilirubin[49]	Acidic	Little clinical significance in dogs Cats—cholestatic disease	
Calcium carbonate[85]	Neutral, alkaline	Not observed in dogs or cats Normal in other species	

Photos	Crystal	pH	Possible Interpretation
	Calcium oxalate dihydrate[38A]	Acidic, neutral, alkaline	Normal Older stored samples artifact Urolithiasis Hyperparathyroidism Miniature Schnauzers are predisposed to the uroliths
	Calcium oxalate monohydrate[38A]	Acidic, neutral, alkaline	Normal Oxalate urolithiasis Hypercalciuric Ethylene glycol toxicity (Picket fence-shaped crystals)

Cystine[10]	Acidic	Defective renal tubular reabsorption; tendency to form uroliths	
Uric (Urate) acid[49]	Acidic	Liver disease Portosystemic shunts Dalmatians and English Bulldogs being predisposed to urate urolithiasis	

COMMON PARASITE PREVENTION RECOMMENDATIONS[92A]

	Less Than 8 Weeks of Age	Over 8 Weeks of Age	6 Months of Age and Older
Internal parasite fecal flotation testing	Four times in the first year of life		Biannually
Tick-transmitted pathogen testing			Annually
Heartworm testing: Antigen and microfilaria			Annually
Heartworm and internal parasite, flea and tick prevention products	Deworm for internal parasites every 2 weeks starting at 2 weeks of age.	Administer year-round broad-spectrum parasite control. Continue even if pregnant and nursing using a product that is appropriately labeled (follow label directions for ages in which products can be started).	

PARASITE IDENTIFICATION AND TREATMENT

Photos	Common Name	Name	Treatment	Dog Dose	Cat Dose
ZOONOTIC	Ascarid Roundworm	Toxocara canis Toxocara leonine	Fenbendazole	50 mg/kg PO q 24 hr × 3 days	50 mg/kg PO q 24 hr × 3 days
			Pyrantel	5–10 mg/kg PO	10–20 mg/kg PO
ZOONOTIC	Hookworm[73]	Ancylostoma Uncinaria	Fenbendazole	50 mg/kg PO q 24 hr × 3 days	100 mg/kg PO
			Ivermectin	0.05 mg/kg SQ or PO	
			Milbemycin oxime	0.5 mg/kg PO	
			Pyrantel	5–10 mg/kg PO	20–30 mg/kg PO

Continued

Photos	Common Name	Name	Treatment	Dog Dose	Cat Dose
	Whipworm[74]	Trichuris Uncinaria	Fenbendazole Ivermectin Milbemycin	50 mg/kg PO q 24 hr × 3 days 0.5 mg/kg SQ or PO 0.5 mg/kg PO	
ZOONOTIC	Tapeworm[75]	Taenia	Fenbendazole Praziquantel	50 mg/kg PO q 24 hr × 3 days 2.5–5 mg/kg PO	2.5–5 mg/kg PO or SQ
	Flea Tapeworm[76]	Diplydium	Praziquantel and Treat for fleas	2.5–5 mg/kg PO	

ZOONOTIC					
	Giardia[107]		Metronidazole	50–70 mg/kg PO q 24 hr × 5 days	25 mg/kg PO q 12 hr × 5 days
	Giardia		Albendazole	25 mg/kg q 12 hr × 2 days	
			Fenbendazole	50 mg/kg PO q 24 hr × 3 days	
	Coccidia[8]		Amprolium	100–200 mg/kg q 24 hr × 7 days	60–100 mg/kg q 24 hr × 7 days
	Isospora		Sulfadimethoxine	55 mg/kg PO q 24 hr × 10 days	55 mg/kg SID then 27.5 mg/kg SID × 5 days

Continued

143

Photos	Common Name	Name	Treatment	Dog Dose	Cat Dose
	Biting louse	Trichodectes	Most topical flea and tick preventatives		
	Sucking louse	Linognathus	Most topical flea and tick preventatives		
	Rodent bot fly[106]	Cuterebra	Careful extraction of larvae and wound treatment		
	Mange[108]	Sarcoptes scabiei Notoedres (Cat)	Ivermectin	0.2 mg/kg PO	
			Selamectin	6–12 mg/kg topically	
			Lime/sulfur dip		

	Follicular mange	Demodex	Milbemycin	2 mg/kg SID × 3 months	Acarexx Milbemite Otomite Plus Selamectin—topically Tresederm (off label)
	Ear mite	Otodectes	Ivermectin	0.6 mg/kg SID until resolved	
	Walking dander	Cheyletiella	Ivermectin		0.3 mg/kg twice at 5-week interval Lime sulfur dip

HEARTWORM/FLEA AND TICK PREVENTIVES FOR DOGS

Product	Active Ingredient	Fleas	Ticks	Heartworms	Mosquitoes	Hookworms	Roundworms	Tapeworms	Whipworms	Notes
Sentinel Spectrum	Milbemycin oxime Lufenuron Praziquantel	◆		◆		◆	◆	◆	◆	
Sentinel Spectrum	Milbemycin oxime Lufenuron Praziquantel	◆		◆		◆	◆	◆	◆	
Advantage Multi (Topical)	Imidacloprid Moxidectin	◆		◆		◆	◆		◆	
Sentinel Flavor Tabs	Milbemycin oxime Lufenuron	◆		◆		◆			◆	

Product	Active Ingredient(s)								Scabies / Ear mites
Sentinel Flavor Tabs	Milbemycin oxime, Lufenuron	◆			◆		◆		◆	
Trifexis Tablet		◆			◆		◆			
Simparica Trio Chewables	Sarolaner, Moxidectin, Pyrantel	◆	◆		◆		◆	◆		
Revolution (Topical)	Selamectin	◆			◆				◆	Scabies / Ear mites
Interceptor Plus Chewable	Milbemycin oxime, Praziquantel	◆			◆	◆	◆		◆	
Heartgard Plus (Chewable)	Ivermectin, Pyrantel				◆		◆	◆		
Interceptor Tabs	Milbemycin oxime	◆			◆		◆			

Continued

147

Product	Active Ingredient	Fleas	Ticks	Heartworms	Mosquitoes	Hookworms	Roundworms	Tapeworms	Whipworms	Notes
Tri Heart Plus Chewable	Ivermectin Pyrantel			◆		◆	◆			
Iverhart Max Chewable	Ivermectin Pyrantel Praziquantel			◆		◆	◆	◆		
Iverhart Plus Flavored Chewables	Ivermectin Pyrantel			◆		◆	◆			
ProHeart 6 and 12 Injectable	Moxidectin			◆		◆				

Product	Active Ingredients					Indications
Frontline Shield for Dogs	Fipronil Permethrin Pyriproxyfen	◆	◆	◆	◆	Flies Lice Scabies
K-9 Advantix II	Imidacloprid Permethrin Pyriproxyfen		◆	◆	◆	Flies Lice
Vectra 3D (Topical)	Dinotefuran Pyriproxyfen Permethrin		◆	◆	◆	Flies Mites (Does not cover mange mites)
Seresto Collar	Flumethrin Imidacloprid			◆	◆	Lice Sarcoptes scabiei
Frontline Gold for Dogs (Topical)	Fipronil Methoprene Pyriproxygen			◆	◆	Lice

Product	Active Ingredient	Fleas	Ticks	Heartworms	Mosquitoes	Hookworms	Roundworms	Tapeworms	Whipworms	Notes
Frontline Spray	Fipronil	◆	◆							Lice Scabies
Nexgard Chewables	Afoxolaner	◆	◆							
Credelio Tablet	Lotilaner	◆	◆							
Bravecto 1 mo Chews	Fluralaner	◆	◆							
Bravecto Chews 3 mo	Fluralaner	◆	◆							
Bravecto Topical	Fluralaner	◆	◆							

							Lice
Simparica Chewables	Sarolaner						◆
Advantage II for Dogs (Topical)	Imidacloprid Pyriproxyfen						◆
Vectra (Topical)	Dinotefuran Pyriproxygen						◆
Comfortis Chewable	Spinosad						◆

The diamond indicates that the product is labeled to treat or prevent those species.

HEARTWORM/FLEA AND TICK PREVENTATIVES FOR CATS

Product	Active Ingredient	Fleas	Ticks	Heartworms	Mosquitoes	Hookworms	Roundworms	Ear Mites	Notes
Advantage Multi for Cats (Topical)	Imidacloprid Moxidectin	◆		◆		◆	◆	◆	
Revolution Plus for Cats (Topical)	Selamectin Sarolaner	◆	◆	◆		◆	◆	◆	
Centragard for Cats (Topical)	Eprinomectin Praziquantel			◆		◆	◆		
Interceptor Flavor Tabs	Milbemycin oxime			◆		◆	◆		
Heartgard Chewables	Ivermectin			◆		◆			

Product	Active Ingredients								Lice
Frontline Gold for Cats (Topical)	Fipronil (S)-Methoprene Pyriproxyfen				◆	◆			Lice
Frontline Spray	Fipronil					◆			Lice
Bravecto Plus for Cats (Topical)	Fluralaner Moxidectin					◆	◆		
Seresto Collar	Flumethrin Imidacloprid					◆	◆		
Vectra for Cats and Kittens	Dinotefuran Pyriproxyfen					◆			
Comfortis Chewable	Spinosad					◆			
Credelio CAT	Lotilaner					◆			
Advantage II (Topical)	Imidacloprid Pyriproxygen					◆			

The diamond indicates that the product is labeled to treat or prevent those species.

CYTOLOGY

Cytology

DTM FUNGAL CULTURE IDENTIFICATION

Photo	Organism	Colony Appearance	Media Color Change
	Microsporum[55]	White, light yellow, tan, or buff-colored, cottony-to-powdery	May not change the media red
	Trichophyton[55]	White, light yellow, tan, or buff-colored, cottony-to-powdery	Red

Note: Environmental fungi can turn the media red.

CHARACTERISTICS OF TUMOR TYPES[51]

Photos	Tumor Type	Cell Shape	Examples
	Epithelial[18]	Large, round to polygonal cells. Distinct cell borders. Tightly adherent to each other. Round to oval nuclei that can be basilar in columnar cells or eccentric in other cell shapes.	Benign = (adenoma) Malignant = (carcinoma)

Continued

Photos	Tumor Type	Cell Shape	Examples
	Mesenchymal[18]	Spindle, oval, or stellate-shaped cells. Indistinct cell borders that taper into the background. Round to oval to elongate nuclei that are usually centrally located. Cells are scattered individually or in aggregates, usually within matrix.	Benign = ("...oma") Malignant = ("sarcoma")

	Mast cell tumor		
	Round cell mast cell tumor[102]	Less cellular than the other tumors due to matrix. Matrix can be present in the background as well as within aggregates. These are readily recognized by the presence of purple cytoplasmic granules. They also have round eccentric nuclei with smooth chromatin.	 10 μm

Continued

Photos	Tumor Type	Cell Shape	Examples
	Round cell histiocytoma[90]	Round to oval with variably distinct cytoplasmic borders. Moderate to abundant amounts of clear to light blue cytoplasm. Nuclei are eccentric and round to oval to indented. Nuclei have finely stippled chromatin, and nucleoli are not apparent. Cells are often found dispersed within a moderately blue background. Minimal cellular atypia, uniform cell size, and morphology—they have a bland appearance.	Histiocytoma

Contin ued

	Plasmacytoma
Round cell plasmacytoma[90]	Round to slightly oval cells. Distinct cell borders. Variable amounts of blue cytoplasm (often deep blue), some have perinuclear clear zones. Nuclei are round, occasionally oval, and eccentric. Nuclei have clumped chromatin and nucleoli are not apparent. More atypia (anisocytosis and anisokaryosis) than histiocytic tumors. Binucleation and, occasionally, multinucleation are common. Multinucleated cells may show marked intracellular anisokaryosis Amyloid may be present in skin tumors.

Photos	Tumor Type	Cell Shape	Examples
	Round cell lymphoma[90]	Lymphoma is most easily recognized when it consists of large cells or cells that are not expected in inflammatory lesions, such as many granular lymphocytes. It is far harder to recognize when the cells are intermediate to small; however, the lack of other immune cells (plasma cells) or inflammatory cells can lead to a suspected diagnosis of lymphoma. Lymphoid cells have the highest nuclear to cytoplasmic ratios of all the round cells.	Lymphoma

Continued

		They can rupture easily and one can see cytoplasmic fragments ("lymphoglandular" bodies) in the background, which can be a helpful but not definitive finding.	Transmissible veneral tumor
	Round cell transmissible veneral tumor[90]	Monomorphic population of round cells. Medium to large round nucleus that is eccentric or central. Nuclear chromatin is clumped and mitotic figures are common. Can see binucleation or multinucleation as well as nucleoli.	

Photos	Tumor Type	Cell Shape	Examples
		The cytoplasm is characteristic: abundant light blue to gray with moderate to many discrete margined vacuoles. Can have infiltrates of small lymphocytes.	Transmissible veneral tumor
	Lipoma	Fails to dry once smeared out on the slide.	Lipoma

COMMON CELL TYPES IN CYTOLOGY SAMPLES

Photos	Sample Type	Description
	Suppurative inflammation[46]	Suppurative inflammation as evidenced by the large number of neutrophils. Note the presence of karyorrhexis in the center cell.
	Pyogranulomatous inflammation[18]	Pyogranulomatous inflammation in the eyelid of a dog. Note neutrophils and epithelioid macrophages, including binucleate forms. Lymphocytes and low numbers of red blood cells also are present.

Continued

Photos	Sample Type	Description
	Septic inflammation[18]	Septic neutrophilic inflammation. Many neutrophils are present, some of which contain phagocytized bacterial rods (arrows).
	Pyogranulomatous lymphadenitis[46]	

| 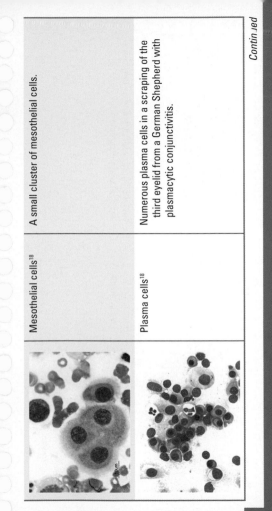 | Mesothelial cells[18] | A small cluster of mesothelial cells. |
| | Plasma cells[18] | Numerous plasma cells in a scraping of the third eyelid from a German Shepherd with plasmacytic conjunctivitis. |

Photos	Sample Type	Description
	Small lymphocytes[85]	Similar in appearance to the small lymphocyte seen on a peripheral blood film. Slightly larger than an RBC. Scanty cytoplasm, dense nucleus.
	Intermediate lymphocytes[85]	Nucleus approximately twice as large as an RBC; abundant cytoplasm.

	Lymphoblasts[49]	Two to four times as large as the RBC. Usually contains a nucleolus. Diffuse nuclear chromatin.
	Plasmablasts[89]	Similar to lymphoblasts with more abundant, basophilic cytoplasm. May contain vacuoles.

Continued

Photos	Sample Type	Description
	Histiocytes[85,111]	Large, pleomorphic, single, or multinuclear; nuclei are round to oval.
	Mast cells[85]	Round cells that usually slightly larger than lymphoblasts; distinctive purple staining granules may not stain adequately with Diff-Quick.

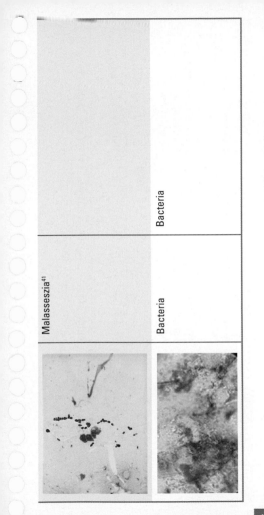

Malasseszia[41]

Bacteria

Bacteria

CHARACTERISTICS OF FLUID SAMPLES[51]

Transudate	Exudate	Normal	Modified Transudate
Origin			
Noninflammatory hypoalbuminemia Vascular stasis Neoplasia	Inflammatory Infection Necrosis		Feline infectious peritonitis Chylous effusion Lymphatic fluid
Amount of Fluid			
Large	Variable	Small	Variable
Color			
Clear, colorless, or red tinged	Turbid, white, slightly yellow	Clear, colorless	Variable, usually clear

Protein			
<3.0 g/dL	>3.0 g/dL	<2.5 g/dL	2.5–7.5 g/dL
TNCC			
<1500/mL	>5000/mL	<3000/mL	1000–7000/mL
Cell Types			
Mixture of monocytes, macrophages, lymphocytes, and mesothelial cells[a] (normal and/or reactive)	Inflammatory: neutrophils, macrophages, lymphocytes,[a] and eosinophils[a]	Same as transudate	Lymphocytes, nondegenerate neutrophils, mesothelial cells, macrophages, and neoplastic cells

[a]Variable numbers.

VAGINAL CYTOLOGY INTERPRETATION

Photos	Cells	Interpretation
	Parabasal cells[18]	Parabasal cells in a vaginal smear from a dog in anestrus.
	Intermediate vaginal epithelial cells[18]	Degenerating superficial vaginal epithelial cells with vacuolated cytoplasm in a canine vaginal smear.

10.0 µm

	Squamous cell[18]	Mature squamous cells have cornified cytoplasm that has sharp angular borders. Mature squamous cells may be nucleated or anucleate. (A) Mature nucleated squamous cells have abundant light blue-gray cytoplasm that has an angular appearance. (B) Mature squamous cell with a pyknotic nucleus (*lower left*) and anucleate, mature squamous cells.
	Cornified cells[18] = 80% or greater reveals cytological estrus. Confirm appropriate breeding time with progesterone.	Mature, cornified cells from a canine vaginal swab. Low-magnification image shows that these cells tend to exfoliate individually rather than in cohesive clusters. Individual cells show angular cytoplasmic borders. Nuclei become pyknotic (*arrow*) and eventually disappear, leaving anucleate cells.

Continued

Photos	Cells	Interpretation
	Natural breeding: should occur 3 days after progesterone reaches 2.5 ng/mL. Chilled semen insemination: breed 48 hr after the progesterone reaches 5 ng/mL. Frozen semen insemination: breed 72 hr after the progesterone reaches 5 ng/mL.	

EMERGENCY AND PROCEDURES

EMERGENCIES

EMERGENCY MEDICATIONS

Dog Emergency Medication Chart[91A]

	Weight in pounds (lb)									
Weight (lb)	5	10	20	30	40	50	60	70	80	90	100
	Weight in kilograms (kg)									
Weight (kg)	2.27	4.55	9.09	13.64	18.18	22.73	27.27	31.82	36.36	40.91	45.45
Drug (conc.)	Amount listed below in milliliter (mL)									
Epinephrine emergency (1:1000) low dose	0.025	0.05	0.10	0.15	0.20	0.25	0.30	0.35	0.40	0.45	0.50
Epinephrine (1:1000) high dose	0.25	0.50	1.00	1.50	2.0	2.50	3.0	3.50	4.0	4.50	5.0

Atropine (0.54 mg/mL)	0.25	0.50	1.00	1.50	2.0	2.50	3.0	3.50	4.0	4.50	5.0
Lidocaine (20 mg/mL)	0.25	0.50	1.00	1.50	2.0	2.50	3.0	3.50	4.0	4.50	5.0
Bicarb (1 mEq/mL)	2.5	5.0	10.0	15.0	20.0	25.0	30.0	35.0	40.0	45.0	50.0
Calcium (100 mg/mL)	1.0	2.50	5.0	7.50	10.0	12.50	15.0	17.50	20.0	22.50	25.0
Magnesium (4 mEq/mL)	0.10	0.25	0.50	0.75	1.00	1.25	1.50	1.75	2.00	2.25	2.50
Vasopressin (20 units/mL)	0.10	0.20	0.40	0.6	0.8	1.0	1.20	1.40	1.60	1.80	2.0

Continued

Dog Emergency Medication Chart[91A]

Reversal agents	Amount listed below in milliliter (mL)										
Amiodarone (50 mg/mL)	0.25	0.50	1.00	1.50	2.00	2.50	3.00	3.50	4.00	4.50	5.00
Naloxone (0.4 mg/mL)	0.25	0.50	1.00	1.50	2.00	2.50	3.00	3.50	4.00	4.50	5.00
Flumazenil (0.1 mg/mL)	0.50	1.0	2.0	3.0	4.0	5.0	6.0	7.0	8.0	9.0	10.0

Doxapram: 1–5 mg **per pup** SC, sublingual or via umbilical vein; repeat in 15–20 min prn. Stimulation of respiration under anesthesia: 5.5–11 mg/kg intravenous (IV); repeat in 15–20 min prn.

Cat Emergency Medication Chart[91A]

					Weight in pounds (lb)					
Weight (lb)	2.2	4.4	6.6	8.8	11	13.2	15.4	17.6	19.8	22.0
					Weight in kilograms (kg)					
Weight (kg)	1	2	3	4	5	6	7	8	9	10
Drug (conc)					Amount listed below in milliliter (mL)					
Epinephrine (1:1000) low dose	0.10	0.10	0.10	0.10	0.10	0.20	0.20	0.20	0.20	0.20
Atropine (0.54 mg/mL)	0.04	0.07	0.11	0.15	0.19	0.22	0.26	0.30	0.33	0.37
Lidocaine (20 mg/mL)	0.01	0.02	0.03	0.04	0.05	0.06	0.07	0.08	0.09	1.0
Sodium bicarbonate (1 mEq/mL)	1.0	2.0	3.0	4.0	5.0	6.0	7.0	8.0	9.0	10.0

Continued

Cat Emergency Medication Chart[91A]

	0.10	0.20	0.30	0.40	0.50	0.60	0.70	0.80	0.90	1.0
Calcium chloride (100 mg/mL)	0.15	0.30	0.45	0.50	0.60	0.75	0.90	1.2	1.35	1.5
Magnesium chloride (4 mEq/mL)										
Amount listed below in milliliter (mL)										
Reversal agents										
Yohimbine (2 mg/mL)	0.07	0.13	0.18	0.25	0.32	0.38	0.44	0.50	1.13	1.25
Naloxone (0.4 mg/mL)	0.08	0.15	0.23	0.30	0.38	0.45	0.53	0.60	0.68	0.75
Flumazenil (0.1 mg/mL)	0.1	0.2	0.3	0.4	0.5	0.6	0.7	0.8	0.9	1.0

Atipamezole (as a reversal for medetomidine): Give the same amount (in mL) as medetomidine.

Dopamine: 1–3 mcg/kg/min.

Doxapram: 1–5 mg **per pup** SC, sublingual or via umbilical vein; repeat in 15–20 min prn. Stimulation of respiration under anesthesia: 5.5–11 mg/kg IV; repeat in 15–20 min prn.

EMERGENCY EVALUATION

Airway	**Cannot breathe**	Ambu bag
		Place endotracheal tube
		Suction airway if needed
		Emergency tracheostomy
	Ventilate with 100% oxygen	Rate of 20–30 per minute
Cardiovascular	**Hypovolemic and circulatory shock**	IV catheterization
	Pale mucus membranes	Blood pressure monitoring
	Prolonged capillary refill time (CRT)>3 sec	
	Weak thready pulses	
	Elevated heart rate	
	Vasodilatory shock	
	Injected mucus membranes	
	Prolonged CRT>1 sec	
	Bounding pulses	

Continued

ECG evaluation		
No pulse or heart rate		External chest compressions at a rate of 80–120 beats per minute Compress abdomen with a sandbag Open-chest cardiac massage
Ventricular asystole[79]		Epinephrine (0.02 mg/kg) Atropine (0.04 mg/kg)
Ventricular fibrillation[80]		Defibrillate 2–4 J
Bradycardia		Atropine (0.4 mg/kg)

		Dog lidocaine (3 mg/kg)
		Cat lidocaine (0.5 mg/kg)
Control pain	**Ventricular tachycardia**[80]	Hydromorphone (0.05 mg/kg)
		Morphine (0.5 mg/kg)
		Oxymorphone (0.05 mg/kg)
Post control	**Lack of consciousness in 15–30 min**	Mannitol (500 mg/kg)
	Arrest greater than 20 min	Dexamethasone (0.5 mg/kg)
		Lasix (5 mg/kg)
		Hyperventilate

185

FLUID THERAPY CALCULATIONS[37]

Calculations of fluid requirements	Bodyweight (kg) × % dehydration = mL of fluid deficit (60 − 80 mL/kg) × bodyweight (kg) = mL of daily fluid requirement EXAMPLE: Bodyweight (kg) × %dehydration × 1000 = mL of fluid deficit (60–80 mL/kg) × bodyweight (kg) = mL of daily fluid requirement Estimation of ongoing losses × 2 = mL of ongoing losses Example: 20kg dog, 8% dehydrated, 100 mL vomitus $20\,kg \times 0.08 \times 1000 = 1600\,mL$ $20\,kg \times 60\,mg/kg = 1200\,mL$ $100\,mL \times 2 = 200\,mL$ Total volume = 3000 mL/24 = 125 mL/hr
Free-drip calculations	$$\text{Drops per minute} = \frac{\text{Total infusion volume} \times \text{drops/mL}}{\text{Total infusion time (min)}}$$
Shock dose	Canine: 80–90 mL/kg Feline: 40–60 mL/kg Administer 1/4–1/3 of calculated dose as bolus. Reassess every 5–10 min and administer additional boluses as needed.

OPHTHALMOLOGY[33]

Best when possible to perform all of the following tests when safe: Schirmer tear test (STT), fluorescein stain, and Intraocular Pressure (IOP); check orbit for foreign bodies.

Name	Common Etiologies	Clinical Signs	Diagnosis	Treatment
Simple superficial ulcer	Trauma Ectopic cilia Foreign body Entropion		Fluorescein stain (only the epithelial layer is damaged)	E-Collar Corneal debridement Antibiotics Atropine for pain applied q 12–24 hr to effect DO NOT USE STEROIDS
Stromal ulcer	Trauma		Fluorescein stain (ulcer with loss of varying amounts of corneal stroma)	E-Collar Antibiotics Atropine for pain applied q 12–24 hr to effect ± *Serum* DO NOT USE STEROIDS

Indolent ulcer	Trauma seems to be more prevalent in older patients		Fluorescein stain (ulcer in which the epithelium will not adhere to the stroma)	E-Collar Corneal debridement Antibiotics Atropine for pain applied q 12–24 hr to effect Diamond bit or grid keratotomy DO NOT USE STEROIDS
Melting ulcer	Severe infection Steroid use		Fluorescein stain (softening and necrosis of the cornea, often associated with infection)	E-Collar Antibiotics ±Serum Atropine for pain applied q 12–24 hr to effect DO NOT USE STEROIDS

Continued

Name	Common Etiologies	Clinical Signs	Diagnosis	Treatment
Descemetocele center is black	Trauma Failure to treat		**Fluorescein stain** (loss of all stromal layers down to Descemet's membrane)	EMERGENCY Transfer immediately to ophthalmologist Use extreme care, do not test handle or restrain the patient further **Conjunctival graft**
Keratoconjunctivitis sicca (KCS) dry eye	Immune-mediated Iatrogenic (drugs and removal of lacrimal gland)	Ocular discharge, conjunctival hyperemia, and chemosis Blepharospasm Dry/lack luster to cornea Corneal vascularization and pigmentation	Clinical signs and STT Corneal ulcers are common secondary disease	**Cyclosporine-A** or tacrolimus DO NOT stop treatment if working

Anterior uveitis	Infectious Chronic eye disease Idiopathic anterior uveitis (cataracts) Or systemic disease	Periocular dermatitis Photophobia	Look for systemic disease IOP is usually low Poor pupillary light reflex (PLR)	*Treat underlying diseases* Topical mydriatics and antiinflammatories
Glaucoma	Increased intraocular fluid production	Ocular pain Corneal edema Buphthalmus blindness Corneal edema Episcleral hyperemia	*Increased tonometry* Pressure	Timolol Dorzolamide Enucleation if not controlled

Continued

Name	Common Etiologies	Clinical Signs	Diagnosis	Treatment
Chalazion and stye (hordeolum)	Infection or gland obstruction	Focal eyelid inflammation or mass	Visual and fine-needle aspirate	Scalpel incision of overlying palpebral conjunctiva with curettage; heals by second intention
Pannus (chronic superficial keratitis)	Immune-mediated disease, ultraviolet radiation exposure at high altitude potentiates the disorder	Nonulcerative, pinkish-red, and/or pigmentary superficial corneal lesions commencing in the lateral to ventrolateral cornea; progressively involving the medial, ventral, and dorsal aspects of the cornea, including the central cornea	Visual Diagnosis. Diagnosis of exclusion all other tests will be negative	Topical corticosteroids Cyclosporine-A Tacrolimus Lifelong therapy

- Ensure all patients with dermatology problems are on flea and tick preventative for 3 months before ruling out fleas or flea allergy.
- Recommend to always perform dermatophyte testing medium (DTM), Wood's lamp, skin scrape, impression smears, and trichogram.

Name	Common Etiologies	Clinical Signs	Diagnosis	Treatment
Fleas and flea allergy	Hypersensitivity to *Ctenocephalides* infestation	Pruritus, alopecia, dermatitis	Visual fleas Apply flea and tick product for 3 months before you can rule out	Flea prevention and treatment
Allergic dermatitis	Food allergy Environmental allergy	Porphyrin staining on feet Licking feet Alopecia Lichenification Pruritus Self-trauma, redness, and secondary skin changes	Rule out all other causes VARL Dermal testing	*Treat secondary infections* Desensitization injections Consider 8- to 12-week food trial to rule out food allergy first, unless seasonal Cyclosporine Apoquel Cytopoint

Acne	Unknown Local trauma Genetic predisposition Poor grooming habits Stress Viruses	Secondary infections Papular dermatitis with alopecia Papular dermatitis with alopecia Typically, on the chin	Cytology Skin scrape—rule out parasites	Prednisone None of the medications will work in the face of secondary infections. Prednisone will always work Chlorhexidine wipes Shampoos

Continued

Name	Common Etiologies	Clinical Signs	Diagnosis	Treatment
Acral lick granuloma	Hypersensitivity, skin disease, pyoderma, joint disease, neoplasia Obsessive–compulsive behavior associated with boredom and separation anxiety	Generally, only a single lesion A firm, erythematous, alopecic, eroded, or ulcerated plaque or nodule Porphyrin staining	Rule out other causes Then visual	E-Collar or basket muzzle Treat secondary infections Treat inflammation Behavior medication Pain medication
Acute moist dermatitis/ hot spot/ moist eczema/ pyotraumatic dermatitis	Scratching or itching	Acute onset of well-demarcated red, moist, and alopecic area that exudes serum and becomes matted with hair, especially at the periphery	Rule out causes other than allergic dermatitis	Clip and clean Treat inflammation Treat secondary infections Control underlying problem

Nasodigital hyperkeratosis	Failure of keratin to wear away during frequent contact	Visual—if no other signs of illness	Lifelong treatment is required Excess keratin may be trimmed Soak in warm water and then apply petroleum jelly once daily for 10 days; weekly application of petroleum jelly and trimming are required to prevent further buildup. Fissures or ulceration may require antiinflammatories or secondary infection treatment

Continued

Name	Common Etiologies	Clinical Signs	Diagnosis	Treatment
Pyoderma (deep)	Bacterial infection of the skin	Papules Pustules Draining fistulous tracts	Cytology Skin scrape to rule out other causes Appearance Culture	Consider allergies as an underlying problem Antibiotics Antiinflammatories Treat underlying problem if suspected
Dermatophytosis ZOONOSIS	Microsporum canis, M. gypseum, or Trichophyton mentagrophytes	Circular area of alopecia; lesion may be raised, red, and crusty	DTM Wood's lamp	Owner wears gloves Topical antifungal Systemic antifungal Tx environment
Pemphigus complex	Autoimmune	Crusts, scabs Pustules Nose Eyes Ears	Biopsy	Immunosuppressive medications

Color dilution alopecia	Genetic	Alopecia in dilute colors	Finding macromelanosomes under microscope	Melatonin control secondary infections

Name	Common Etiologies	Clinical Signs	Diagnosis	Treatment
Eosinophilic granuloma complex	Possibly allergic or infectious—unknown	Raised lesions tongue, lips (rodent ulcers), and feet	Biopsy	Steroids Cyclosporine Tx secondary infections
Seborrheic dermatitis	Primary or secondary	Excessive scaling or greasy skin	Appearance	Shampoo
Juvenile cellulitis	Unknown	Acute swelling of the face Lymphadenopathy Pustules for on face within 48 hr	Clinical signs	Prednisone and antibiotics
Cat fight abscess	Cat scratches and bites	Abscess with scratches or puncture wounds	Visual	Lance/drain/flush Antibiotics Pain medication

OTIC

Note: It is always recommended to perform cytology. Always check to see if the tympanic membrane is ruptured or intact.

Name	Common Etiologies	Clinical Signs	Diagnosis	Treatment
Otitis externa	Allergies Immune mediated Parasites Plucking hair Parasitic, bacterial, or yeast infection of the soft tissues of the ear	Head shaking Head tilt Pain Foul odor	*Cytology* Culture	**Clean the ears first!** Treat parasites if present Antibiotics and antinflammatories Treat the underlying disease
Otitis interna/ media	Extension of otitis externa	Vestibular disease Facial paralysis Horner's syndrome	Rule out other causes	Systemic and local antibiotics Pain medication Antiinflammatory Myringotomy Ventral or lateral bulla osteotomy

Continued

Name	Common Etiologies	Clinical Signs	Diagnosis	Treatment
Aural hematoma	Trauma causing buildup of blood beneath skin surface	Head shaking Scratching at ear	 Visual	Surgery

DENTAL

Name	Common Etiologies	Clinical Signs	Diagnosis	Treatment
Periodontal disease	Bacterial infection of tissues surrounding teeth that leads to plaque accumulation and causes calculus buildup	Increased depth of periodontal pockets Increased tooth mobility Foul oral odor Pain	Visual Dental radiography	Comprehensive Oral Health Assessment and Treatment (COHAT)
Abscess	Infection	Facial swelling Regional lymphadenitis	Dental radiology	Extraction Antibiotics Pain medications
Fracture	Trauma	Fractured tooth	Visual	If pulp exposure, extraction

Continued

Name	Common Etiologies	Clinical Signs	Diagnosis	Treatment
Epulide	Tumor	Local, exophytic growth on the gingiva	Biopsy	Surgery
Persistent deciduous teeth	Abnormal dental development	Retained baby teeth	Visual	Extraction
Feline gingivostomatitis	Immune mediated	Gingivitis	Visual	Antibiotics Steroids Extractions
Feline oral resorptive lesions	Multiple	Tooth resorption on dental radiology	Dental radiology	Extraction

Name	Common Etiologies	Clinical Signs	Diagnosis	Treatment
Viral rhinotracheitis (feline)	Herpesvirus infection	Sneezing Conjunctivitis purulent rhinitis Fever	Visual	Antiviral Lysine Tx secondary infection
Calicivirus (feline)	Viral infection of upper respiratory tract	Anorexia Lethargy Fever Ulcerative stomatitis Nasal discharge	Visual	Antiviral Tx secondary infection
Brachycephalic respiratory distress syndrome	Congenital airway obstruction	Coughing Exercise intolerance Cyanosis Dyspnea	Visual	Surgery

Continued

Name	Common Etiologies	Clinical Signs	Diagnosis	Treatment
Infectious canine tracheobronchitis (kennel cough)	Bacterial and viral infection of lower respiratory tract (*Bordetella bronchiseptica*, canine adenovirus, etc.)	Dry, hacking, paroxysmal cough	History Clinical Signs Vaccination status	Doxycycline or other antibiotics
Reverse sneeze	Normal or reflex from disease	Sneezing that almost appears inward	Look for underlying problem, solve underlying problem	**Occasional, do nothing** Treat underlying problem if present

| Tracheal collapse | Unknown | Recurrent loud, honking cough Gagging or retching | I: <25% reduction in diameter; generally not associated with clinical signs
• II: 50% reduction in airway lumen, tracheal rings elongated and mildly flattened
• III: 75% reduction in airway lumen, tracheal rings markedly flattened | Cough suppressants, antiinflammatory medication, bronchodilators, and, in severe cases, surgical treatment |

Continued

Name	Common Etiologies	Clinical Signs	Diagnosis	Treatment
			• IV: >90% reduction in airway lumen, severely flattened tracheal rings, possibly with dorsal deviation of ventral tracheal surface; generally associated with frequent, constant, or severe clinical signs	
Bronchitis sterile	Aging dogs	Dry, hacking cough	Radiographs	Bronchodilator Antiinflammatories and cough suppressants

				Bronchodilators Steroids
Asthma (feline)	Allergic	Dyspnea Coughing Lethargy	Wheezing Radiographs—bronchial or broncho-interstitial pattern	
Diaphragmatic hernia	Trauma	Hypovolemic shock Dyspnea and/or tachypnea Pale or cyanotic mucous membranes Tachycardia Cardiac arrhythmias Muffled heart and lung sounds Borborygmi on thoracic auscultation	Radiographs	Surgery

Continued

Name	Common Etiologies	Clinical Signs	Diagnosis	Treatment
		Tucked-up or empty appearance of the abdomen Abdominal distention with fluid wave if ascites		
Pneumonia	Infection Aspiration	Cough Respiratory distress	Radiographs	Antibiotics Consider antifungal if suspected

CARDIOLOGY

NOTE: It is best practice to recommend all patients receive an echocardiogram.

Name	Common Etiologies	Clinical Signs	Diagnosis	Treatment
Congestive heart failure	Mitral regurgitation Tricuspid regurgitation Aortic stenosis Pulmonic stenosis Aortic insufficiency	Anorexia Syncope Pulmonary edema	Radiographs Vertebral heart score Murmur Resting respiratory rate greater than 30	Furosemide Benazepril or enalapril Spironolactone Pimobendan Monitor resting respiratory rate
Hypertrophic cardiomyopathy	Defect Hyperthyroidism	Murmur Arrhythmia Dyspnea	Radiographs Valentine Heart Confirm echo	Atenolol Angiotensin-converting enzyme inhibitors Clopidogrel

Continued

211

Name	Common Etiologies	Clinical Signs	Diagnosis	Treatment
Heartworm disease	Dirofilaria immitis parasite	Exercise intolerance, dyspnea, coughing Ascites	Antigen test Microfilaria in buffy coat	**See Parasitology** Heartworm Protocol
Pericarditis	Idiopathic Infectious	Tachycardia Muffled heart sounds Thready pulses Jugular distention Abdominal distention Ascites	ECG-electrical alternans Radiographs Ultrasound	Pericardiocentesis Surgery
Patent ductus arteriosus	Developmental	Incidental murmur	Echocardiography	Surgery

GASTROINTESTINAL

Name	Common Etiologies	Clinical Signs	Diagnosis	Treatment
Gastric ulcer	Iatrogenic Kidney failure Gastric disease Shock	Vomiting, hematemesis, and melena Inappetance Abdominal pain	Suspect—Endoscopy	Symptomatic—Omeprazole
Perianal fistula	A genetic and immunologic etiology is suspected	Perianal pain, multiple ulcerated, draining tracts circumferentially extending around the anus Loss of anal tone	Palpation	Clip and clean Remove retained feces Antibiotics Pain medication Immunosuppression

Continued

Name	Common Etiologies	Clinical Signs	Diagnosis	Treatment
Salmon poisoning	*(Neorickettsia helminthoeca)*, and therefore the disease, from a fluke parasite *(Nanophyetus salmincola)*	Acute Febrile 5–7 days after fish ingestion; often fatal	Clinical signs History Fecal floatation	Supportive care Doxycycline Praziquantel
Hemorrhagic gastroenteritis	Unknown	Defecation of what appears to be extremely bloody fecal material	Presumptive Rule out other causes	Fluids Antiemetics Probiotics Antibiotics
Megaesophagus	Congenital Idiopathic	Regurgitation Cough Drooling	Radiographs Acetylcholine receptor antibodies	Check for aspiration pneumonia Feed modification Prokinetic

Portosystemic shunt	Embryonic malfunction	Stunted body size Unthrifty appearance Unique copper-colored iris in cats	Low blood urea nitrogen Ultrasound	Surgery
Triandenitis	Infectious Immune mediated	Anorexia Fever Vomiting	• Leukocytosis; neutrophilia with a left shift and/or toxic neutrophils • Lymphocytosis Mild nonregenerative anemia • Elevated liver enzyme • Possibly elevated total bilirubin concentration	Symptoms Fluids Antibiotics Ursodeoxycholic acid Vitamin K Steroids

Continued

Name	Common Etiologies	Clinical Signs	Diagnosis	Treatment
			• Hyperglobulinemia • High feline pancreatic lipase immunoreactivity (fPLI) possible with pancreatitis • Low-serum cobalamin concentration with severe inflammatory bowel disease • Hepatomegaly	
Intussusception	Unknown	Diarrhea hematochezia Vomiting, anorexia, lethargy, weight loss	Ultrasound	Surgery

GI lymphoma	Cancer	Older cats FeLV negative Anorexia, weight loss, vomiting, diarrhea	Biopsy	Chemotherapy
Gastroenteritis	*Salmonella,* *Escherichia coli*	Diarrhea	Rule out other causes Diagnosis of exclusion	Bland diet Resume feeding slowly Probiotics Antibiotic Antidiarrheal Antiemetic GI protectants Antacids

Continued

Name	Common Etiologies	Clinical Signs	Diagnosis	Treatment
Lymphangiectasia	Unknown	Weight loss Low BCS	Hypoalbuminemia Canine fecal alpha1-proteinase inhibitor	Ultra-low-fat diet Immunosuppressant Clopidogrel Diuretic Antibiotic
Liver disease	Drugs, toxins, bile duct inflammation	Anorexia Vomiting Diarrhea PU/PD Jaundice	Elevated liver enzymes Biopsy Check the gallbladder with ultrasound	SAME Diet Supportive
Hepatic lipidosis	Accumulation of triglycerides in liver	Prolonged anorexia Vomiting Diarrhea Lethargy	Ultrasound	Supplemental nutrition

Parvovirus (canine)	Viral infection of gastrointestinal tract	Bloody diarrhea Lethargy Dehydration Fever	Enzyme-linked immunosorbent assay	Supportive care
Coronavirus	Viral infection of gastrointestinal system	Asymptomatic Anorexia Dehydration Vomiting Diarrhea	Suggestive Rule out other causes	Supportive Antidiarrheal Probiotics
Inflammatory bowel disease	Inflammation of intestinal mucosa	Diarrhea Increased frequency and volume of defecation	Biopsy	Immunosuppressants

Continued

Name	Common Etiologies	Clinical Signs	Diagnosis	Treatment
Peritonitis	Inflammatory process	Abdominal pain Reluctance to move Tachycardia Tachypnea, fever Vomiting Diarrhea Dehydration	CBC chemistry suspect	Supportive care Antibiotics
Renal failure	Damage to nephron causing reduction in glomerular filtration	Oliguria Polyuria Vomiting Diarrhea Anorexia Dehydration	Azotemia Rule out other causes Stage 1: <1.4/<125 <1.6/<140 Stage 2: 1.4–2.0/125–179 1.6–2.8/140–249	Fluids Diet Treat underlying cause if possible Azodyl

| Hepatic abscess | Infection | Lethargy
Anorexia
Abdominal pain
Vomiting
Weight loss
Diarrhea
PU/PD | Ultrasound | Stage 3:
2.1–5.0/180–439
2.9–5.0/250–439
Stage 4:
>5.0/>440
>5.0/>440 | Fluids
Antibiotics
Drain the abscess using FNA |

Continued

Name	Common Etiologies	Clinical Signs	Diagnosis	Treatment
Cholecystitis	Bacterial	Vomiting Diarrhea Depression Weight loss Abdominal pain	Biopsy culture	Surgery
Gallbladder mucocele	Unknown	Vomiting Inappetance Lethargy Weight loss Diarrhea Ptyalism PU/PD	Ultrasound	Surgery

Megacolon/ constipation	Multiple	Lack of defecation or very hard, dry stools	Radiographs Look for underlying cause	Fluids Enemas Antibiotics Stool softeners Prokinetic
Cholecysto-lithiasis	Unknown	Vomiting Anorexia Lethargy Weakness Polydipsia and polyuria Weight loss Icterus	Radiographs Ultrasound	Incidental—no treatment Surgery
Foreign body	Ate something that it should not have	Vomiting	Radiographs	Surgery

Continued

Name	Common Etiologies	Clinical Signs	Diagnosis	Treatment
Gastric dilatation-volvulus	Unknown	Abdominal distention Abdominal pain Ptyalism Retching or vomiting Acute collapse	Radiographs—Smurf Hat	Surgery
Inguinal hernia	Congenital Acquired	Protrusion of abdominal contents into the subcutaneous space through a defect in the inguinal ring(s)	Visual	Surgery

Perianal hernia	Unknown	Weakness and separation of the muscles of the pelvic diaphragm allowing prolapse of tissue/organs	Visual	Surgery
Umbilical hernia	Congenital	Full-thickness abdominal wall defect at the umbilicus	Visual	Surgery
Rectal prolapse	Straining	Eversion of the anal mucosa or full-thickness rectal wall through the anal opening	Visual	Manual reduction Purse string Tx underlying cause of straining

ANAL GLANDS

Name	Common Etiologies	Clinical Signs	Diagnosis	Treatment
Anal sacculitis	Impaction, inflammation, or infection of anal glands	Scooting Tail chewing Malodorous perianal discharge	Visual	Express anal glands Anal gland infusion Flush anal glands Antibiotics
Anal gland rupture	Impaction, inflammation, or infection of anal glands	An open skin wound into the anal sac	Visual	E-Collar Anal gland flush Topical and systemic antibiotics

URINARY TRACT

Name	Common Etiologies	Clinical Signs	Diagnosis	Treatment
Cystitis	Inflammation or bacterial infection of urinary bladder	Hematuria Dysuria, Inappropriate urination Pollakiuria Polyuria	Urinalysis culture	Antibiotics
Urolithiasis	Precipitation of mineral substances in urine	Dysuria Hematuria	Radiographs Ultrasound	Surgery Diet with smal stones
Obstruction	Multiple	Enlarged, turgid urinary bladder Abdominal discomfort Dribbling urine Bloody preputial/vulvar discharge Palpable urethral urolith or tumor Bradycardia	Enlarged firm urinary bladder	Stabilization Urethral catheterization

Continued

Name	Common Etiologies	Clinical Signs	Diagnosis	Treatment
Feline lower urinary tract disease	Idiopathic	Difficult or painful urination Pollakiuria Inappropriate urination	Diagnosis of exclusion	Stress reduction Diet
Estrogen responsive urinary incontinence	Hormonal	Leaking urine while sleeping	History: common in spayed females Rule out neurological	Proin
Benign prostatic hyperplasia	Cysts Tumors	Most common in intact male; if neutered, look for cancer	Rectal examination Radiography	Castration
Prostatitis	Infection	Fever Abdominal pain Urethral discharge	Prostatic fluid cytology	SMZ or enrofloxacin

Name	Common Etiologies	Clinical Signs	Diagnosis	Treatment
Osteoarthritis	Progressive degeneration of hyaline cartilage	Lameness Swelling Crepitus	Crepitus Radiographs	Pain medication Diet Weight loss Joint supplement Adequan Joint Injection
Patellar luxation	Unknown	Patella can be manually displaced into and out of the trochlear groove during flexion and extension with grades 1 and 2 luxations; crepitus may be palpable with grade 2	Physical exam	**See Physical Examination Chapter**

Continued

Name	Common Etiologies	Clinical Signs	Diagnosis	Treatment
CCL rupture	Injury	Unilateral or bilateral hindlimb lameness	Cranial drawer	Surgery under 40 pounds can perform lateral suture and over 40 pounds perform TPLO
Hip dysplasia	Abnormal development	Lameness Gait abnormality Muscle atrophy	Radiographs	Nonsteroidal antiinflammatory drugs (NSAIDS) Maintain low body weight Surgery

| Panosteitis | Possible viral infection, metabolic disease, allergic reaction, hormonal excesses | Young dogs
Intermittent lameness
Anorexia
Fever
Weight loss | Radiographs
Patchy areas of increased intramedullary opacity
• Increased radiographic lucency near the nutrient foramen of the bone
• Increased periosteal bone formation | NSAIDS |

Continued

Name	Common Etiologies	Clinical Signs	Diagnosis	Treatment
Lyme disease	*Borrelia burgdorferi*	Fever Anorexia Lameness Lymphadenopathy	Antibody test	Doxycycline or amoxicillin
Elbow dysplasia	Developmental	Lameness on one or both front limbs	Radiology	Surgery
Fracture	Trauma	Non-weight-bearing lameness	Radiology	Cast Surgery

			Radiology	NSAIDS
Hypertrophic osteodystrophy	Unknown	Fever Swelling Lameness	Pathognomonic lucent line adjacent to the physis on the metaphyseal side ("double physis" or "scorbutic line")	Ensure appropriate diet
Hypertrophic osteopathy	Unknown	Lethargy Low-grade lameness or reluctance to move	Radiographs Fungal disease Panosteitis	Look for cancer

Continued

Name	Common Etiologies	Clinical Signs	Diagnosis	Treatment
Hip luxation	Trauma	Variable lameness Legs are different lengths when the patient is lying on its back	Radiographs	Closed reduction Surgery
Osteomyelitis	Infection	Fever Lethargy Anorexia Limb or joint swelling/pain lameness	Radiographs Biopsy	Antibiotics
Elbow hygroma	Trauma	Soft-tissue swelling, containing serum, that is located between skin and bony prominence (olecranon)	Visual—FNA	Decrease continued trauma

HEMATOLOGY

Name	Common Etiologies	Clinical Signs	Diagnosis	Treatment
Anemia caused by hemorrhage	Trauma	Anorexia Weakness Depression Tachycardia Tachypnea Pale mucous membranes	CBC/blood smear • Normocytic, normochromic RBCs initially • Reticulocytosis occurs 3–5 days after acute loss; hypochromic macrocytosis and polychromasia • Microcytosis, increased red cell distribution width, hypochromasia suggests chronic blood loss/iron-deficiency anemia • Platelet count usually normal	Treat trauma Fluids Blood transfusion

Continued

Name	Common Etiologies	Clinical Signs	Diagnosis	Treatment
Immune-mediated hemolytic anemia	Accelerated red blood cell destruction	Anorexia, depression, tachycardia, tachypnea Pale mucous membranes	Regenerative anemia and normal blood protein concentration are accompanied by spherocytosis (in the absence of recent RBC transfusion) and/or autoagglutination	Immuno-suppressants
Aplastic anemia	Idiopathic most common	Possible mucosal bleeding Pale mucus membranes Tachypnea, tachycardia	CBC: neutropenia, eosinopenia, and thrombocytopenia occur first, followed by moderate-to-severe nonregenerative anemia • Reticulocyte count: corrected count <1%; absolute count <60,000/ mcL	Immuno-suppressive

| Immune-mediated thrombocytopenia | Numerous viral, bacterial, immune-mediated, and other noninfectious causes | Petechiae, ecchymoses
Ocular hemorrhage/hyphema
GI bleeding
Pale mucous membranes
Fever in <20% of cases | Confirmed by demonstrating repeatable, severe thrombocytopenia (<50,000/mcL) in the absence of an identifiable cause | Immuno-suppressive |

Name	Common Etiologies	Clinical Signs	Diagnosis	Treatment
Hyperlipidemia	Primary Secondary	Anorexia Lethargy Vomiting Diarrhea Abdominal discomfort Seizures Cats cutaneous/subcutaneous masses Cats lameness	Increased fasting blood cholesterol and/or triglyceride (TG) concentrations	Dietary management
Hyperthyroidism	Overproduction of thyroid hormone	Weight loss Polyphagia Vomiting Enlarged thyroid	Thyroid test	Felimazole I-131 Iodine-restricted diet Thyroidectomy

Hypothyroidism	Underproduction of thyroid hormone	Weight gain Bilateral, symmetrical alopecia Cold intolerance	Free T4 by ED	Levothyroxine
Diabetes mellitus	Deficient or defective production of insulin	PU/PD Weight loss polyphagia	Blood glucose>200 mg/dL (11 mmol/L) and persistent glycosuria	Diet modification Insulin
Pancreatitis	Inflammation of the pancreas due to obesity, over-ingestion of fats, other diseases	Depression Anorexia Vomiting Diarrhea Dehydration	fPLI or cPLI	Fluids Pain medication Antibiotics

Continued

Name	Common Etiologies	Clinical Signs	Diagnosis	Treatment
Cushing's disease	Hyperadrenocorticism	Bilateral, symmetrical alopecia Potbelly appearance Stress leukogram	LDDT ACTH stim	Trilostane
Addison's disease	Hypoadrenocorticism	Weakness Lethargy Anorexia Vomiting Great mimic	ACTH Stim	DOCP injection or oral fludrocortisone

TICK BORNE

Name	Common Etiologies	Clinical Signs	Diagnosis	Treatment
Ehrlichia canis, E. ewingii, E. equi (ehrlichiosis), Anaplasma platys (anaplasmosis)	*Ehrlichia canis, E. ewingii, E. equi (ehrlichiosis), Anaplasma platys (anaplasmosis)*	Lymphadenopathy Anemia Depression, anorexia Fever Lethargy Lameness, thrombocytopenia, muscular stiffness	Antigen test PCR Thrombocytopenia	Doxycycline
Rocky Mountain Spotted Fever	*Rickettsia rickettsii*	Fever Anorexia Ocular discharge, coughing, tachypnea Vomiting Diarrhea	Antigen PCR Thrombocytopenia	Doxycycline

NEUROLOGY

Name	Common Etiologies	Clinical Signs	Diagnosis	Treatment
Intervertebral disk disease	Trauma Degeneration	Lack of proprioception Lack of motor function Lack of deep pain	Neurological exam Radiographs MRI	Muscle relaxants Steroids
Epilepsy	Unknown	Loss of consciousness and sustained contraction of all muscles, followed by paddling motions of the limbs or rhythmic muscle contractions, especially of the limbs and masticatory muscles	Rule out other causes and syncope Two within a month Status epilepticus lasts longer than 3 minutes	Antiseizure medication

Fibrocartilaginous embolism	Unknown	Neurologic deficits Nociception and proprioception can be affected	Rule out other causes MRI	Supportive care
Old dog vestibular syndrome	Unknown	Head tilt Circling Disorientation Ataxia Nystagmus	Rule out other causes	Supportive care
Myasthenia gravis	Congenital Acquired	Generalized limb weakness Stiffness Tremor Short-strided gait and megaesophagus	Serum ACH antibody levels Radiographs	Pyridostigmine Check for aspiration pneumonia

Continued

Name	Common Etiologies	Clinical Signs	Diagnosis	Treatment
Tick paralysis	Feeding female tick attached	Hindlimb weakness rapidly progressing to generalized weakness, then complete flaccid paralysis Tail wag often is preserved	Ticks with clinical signs	Supportive care Tick removal is curative
Polyradiculoneuritis Coonhound paralysis	Unknown	Nonambulatory LMN paraparesis/plegia or tetraparesis/plegia Normal cognition	Diagnosis of exclusion	Supportive care
Rabies	Virus	Prodromal Paralytic Furious	Necropsy	None

Name	Common Etiologies	Clinical Signs	Diagnosis	Treatment
Lipoma	Benign fatty tumor	Soft and round or oval subcuticular mass	FNA	None required if affecting movement surgery
Skin tumors (sebaceous cysts, adenoma, adenocarcinoma, melanoma)	Unknown; possible genetic causes	Usually round masses, may be encapsulated or ulcerated	Biopsy	Surgery
Mast cell tumor	Tumor	Tumor	FNA-blue- or purple-staining intracytoplasmic granules Biopsy	Surgery Chemotherapy

Continued

Name	Common Etiologies	Clinical Signs	Diagnosis	Treatment
Mammary tumors	Tumor	Mammary tumor	Biopsy: 30%–50% of dogs malignant	Surgery
Squamous cell carcinoma	Tumor	Tends to be face	Biopsy	Surgery Chemotherapy
Hemangiosarcoma	Tumor	Bleeding Exercise intolerance Weight loss	Radiographs Ultrasound Biopsy	Surgery
Viral papilloma	Virus	Benign Tumor Small cauliflower tend to be oral	Biopsy	Spontaneously regress in 2–3 months

Histiocytoma	Benign skin tumor	Fast-growing dome or button-like nodules; may be ulcerated	Biopsy	Spontaneous remission may occur within 3 months. Surgical excision is curative for lesions that do not regress
Transitional cell carcinoma	Tumor	Pollakiuria Hematuria Stranguria	Ultrasound Bladder tumor antigen Cytology	Surgery Chemotherapy
Osteosarcoma	Tumor	Lameness	Radiographs	Surgery

REPRODUCTION

Name	Common Etiologies	Clinical Signs	Diagnosis	Treatment
Dystocia	Primary uterine inertia, fetal obstruction	Active prolonged straining with no fetus produced Green, purulent, or hemorrhagic vaginal discharge	Visual	Obstetrics Fetotomy C-section
Pyometra	Bacterial infection	Vulvar discharge, abdominal enlargement PU/PD, dehydration	Radiographs Ultrasound In heat recently Leukocytosis (HIGH), leukopenia	Spay Antibiotics

		Abdominal enlargement	Radiographs Ultrasound	None
Pregnancy	Normal		Radiographs Ultrasound	None
Mastitis	Infection	Mammary gland inflammation Purulent discharge	Visual Culture	Antibiotics Infusion
Vaginal prolapse	Genetic	Vaginal protrusion through the vulvar lips	*Visual*	Dogs will resolve when heat ends—keep clean
Uterine prolapse	Straining	Protrusion of the uterus	Visual	**DO NOT MOVE** Clean Replace Purse string

Continued

Name	Common Etiologies	Clinical Signs	Diagnosis	Treatment
Eclampsia	Moderate-to-severe hypocalcemia of lactating females, most often occurring in the first 4 weeks postpartum	Anxiety Restlessness, disinterest in puppies Pruritus Ataxia Dyspnea Mydriasis Decreased PLR Tachycardia Bradycardia Muscle tremors Seizures Hyperthermia Arrhythmias	History and clinical signs along with response to treatment	Calcium gluconate

Priapism	Unknown	Persistent penile erection	Physical exam	Hypertonic compress Lubrication Manual reduction
Vaginitis	Unknown	Vaginal discharge Vulvar hyperemia	Suspect	in juveniles will spontaneously resolve

COMMONLY USED MEDICAL PRESCRIPTION ABBREVIATIONS[7]

Abbreviation	Meaning
Bid	twice daily
Disp	dispense
g (or gm)	gram
Gr	grain
Gtt	drop
h (or hr)	hour
IC	intracardiac
IM	intramuscular
IP	intraperitoneal
IV	intravenous
L	liter
Mg	milligram
mL (or mL)	milliliter
OD	right eye
OS	left eye
OU	both eyes
PO	by mouth
Prn	as needed
Q	every
q4h	every 4 hr
Qd	every day (daily)
Qid	four times daily
Qod	every other day

Sid	once a day
SQ (or SC)	subcutaneous
Stat	immediately
TBL or Tbsp	tablespoon
Tid	three times daily
TD	transdermal
TM	transmucosal
Tsp	teaspoon

CONVERSION FACTORS[7]

Weight or Mass
1 kilogram (kg) = 2.2 pounds (lb)
1 kilogram (kg) = 1000 grams (g)
1 kilogram (kg) = 1,000,000 milligrams (mg)
1 gram (g) = 1000 milligrams (mg)
1 gram (g) = 0.001 kilogram (kg)
1 milligram (mg) = 0.001 gram (g)
1 milligram (mg) = 1000 micrograms (μg or mcg)
1 pound (lb) = 0.454 kilogram (kg)
1 pound (lb) = 16 ounces (oz)
1 grain (gr) = 64.8 milligrams (mg) (household system)
1 grain (gr) = 60 milligrams (mg) (apothecary)

Continued

Volume	
1 liter (L) = 1000 milliliters (mL)	
1 liter (L) = 10 deciliters (dL)	
1 milliliter (mL) = 1 cubic centimeter (cc)	
1 milliliter (mL) = 1000 microliters (µL or mcL)	
1 tablespoon (TBL or Tbsp) = 3 teaspoons (tsp)	
1 tablespoon (TBL or Tbsp) = 15 milliliters (mL)	
1 teaspoon (tsp) = 5 milliliters (mL)	
1 gallon (gal) = 3.786 liters (L)	
1 gallon (gal) = 4 quarts (qt)	
1 gallon (gal) = 8 pints (pt)	
1 pint (pt) = 2 cups (c)	
1 pint (pt) = 16 fluid ounces (fl oz)	
1 pint (pt) = 473 milliliters (mL)	

EMPIRICAL THERAPY BY LOCATION PENDING CULTURE

Bone and synovial	Clindamycin Cephalexin Cefadroxil Cefazolin Clavamox Enrofloxacin Marbofloxacin Gentamicin Amikacin
Blood brain and ocular barriers	Doxycycline Metronidazole Trimethoprim-sulfa Enrofloxacin
Gastrointestinal tract	Trimethoprim-sulfa Metronidazole Doxycycline Tetracycline Minocycline Enrofloxacin Ampicillin
Gingivitis/ stomatitis	Clindamycin Metronidazole Tetracycline Clavamox
Hepatobiliary	Cefoxitin Metronidazole Gentamicin Ampicillin Amoxicillin Doxycycline

Continued

Prostate or metritis	Clindamycin Enrofloxacin Marbofloxacin Trimethoprim-sulfa
Septicemia	Aminoglycoside (gentamicin, amikacin, neomycin) + penicillin or cephalosporin
Soft tissue infections and dermatitis	Clavamox Cephalexin Cefovecin Clindamycin Cefazolin Cefadroxil Penicillin Ampicillin Tetracycline Trimethoprim-sulfa
Respiratory tract infections	Doxycycline Cephalexin Clavamox Ampicillin Amikacin Enrofloxacin Gentamicin Trimethoprim-sulfa Clindamycin
Urinary tract infections	Ampicillin Clavamox Cephalexin Trimethoprim-sulfa Enrofloxacin Marbofloxacin

Wounds: contaminated and bite	Clindamycin Clavamox Cefovecin Cephalexin Doxycycline Trimethoprim-sulfa Enrofloxacin +/− Metronidazole
Severe unknown	Clindamycin + enrofloxacin

ANTIMICROBIALS[62A]

Generic Name	Trade Names	Dog Dose	Cat Dose	Notes
Aminoglycosides: Bactericidal—Keep Patient Hydrated; Nephrotoxic, Ototoxic				
Amikacin	Amiglyde-V Amikacin K-9, AmiMax	15–30 mg/kg IM, IV, SC q 24 hr	10–14 mg/kg IM, IV, SC q 24 hr	Intrauterine doses available
Gentamicin	Gentocin, Garasol Numerous	9–14 mg/kg IM, IV, SC q 24 hr	5–8 mg/kg IM, IV, SC q 24 hr	
Neomycin	Abbeyneo, Biosol Keraplex, Neoject Neomed, Neomix Neo-Sol	11 mg/kg IM, IV divided into 3–4 daily doses × 3–5 days SC, PO	11 mg/kg IM, IV divided into 3–4 daily doses × 3–5 days	
Penicillins: Bactericidal				
Amoxicillin	Amoxi-Tabs, Biomo, Robamox-V Numerous	10–20 mg/kg PO q 8 hr	6–22 mg/kg PO q 8 hr	Give with food if GI upset occurs

| Penicillin G sodium | Numerous | 15–25 mg/kg IV, IM q 4–6 hr Penicillin G procaine: 30 mg/kg SQ q 24 hr Penicillin G procaine and benzathine combined: 15 mg/kg Procaine penicillin with 11.25 mg/kg benzathine penicillin equivalent to 1 mL per 10 kg body weight | 15–25 mg/kg IV, IM q 4–6 hr Penicillin G procaine: 30 mg/kg SQ q 24 hr Penicillin G procaine and benzathine combined: 15 mg/kg Procaine penicillin with 11.25 mg/kg benzathine penicillin equivalent to 1 mL per 10 kg body weight | Rapid IV administration may cause seizures |

Continued

Generic Name	Trade Names	Dog Dose	Cat Dose	Notes
Amoxicillin with clavulanic acid	Clavamox Numerous	12.5–25 mg/kg PO q 12 hr	10–20 mg/kg PO q 12 hr	Good for bone and synovial fluid An alternative for bacteria that have developed resistance to amoxicillin Do not use orally in rabbits
Ampicillin	Polyflex Numerous	10–40 mg/kg IM, PO, SC q 8 hr	7–40 mg/kg IM, IV, PO, SC q 8–12 hr	Do not give orally to rabbits Give IV slowly

Ampicillin/sulbactam	Unasyn	15–30 mg/kg IM, IV	15–30 mg/kg IM, IV	Similar activity as clavulanate Give slowly IV Administer deeply IM

Cephalosporins: Bactericidal: Caution in Patients Allergic to Penicillin: Good for Skin, Bone, Brain, CSF, Eyes, and Synovial Fluid

Cefadroxil	Duracef Cefa Cefa-Tabs	11–35 mg/kg PO q 12 hr	22 mg/kg PO q 24 hr	First-generation cephalosporin
Cefazolin	Ancef Kefzol	15–25 mg/kg IM, IV, SC q 4–8 hr	33 mg/kg IM, IV q 8–12 hr	First-generation cephalosporin IV slow

Continued

Generic Name	Trade Names	Dog Dose	Cat Dose	Notes
Cefovecin sodium	Convenia	8 mg/kg SC	8 mg/kg SC	Single injection provides 14-day therapeutic level
Cephalexin	Keflex Celexin Cepexin Cephacillin Ceporexin Rilexine	15–35 mg/kg PO q 12 hr	15–30 mg/kg PO q 12 hr	First-generation cephalosporin
Cefoxitin	Mefoxin Mefoxitin	30 mg/kg IM, IV, SC q 6–8 hr	25–30 mg/kg IM, IV q 8 hr	Second-generation cephalosporin

Cefpodoxime	Cefpoderm Proxetil Simplicef Vantin	5 mg/kg PO q 24 hr 24–42 days	5 mg/kg PO q 24 hr × 24–42 days	Third-generation cephalosporin

Tetracyclines: Bacteriostatic—Can Cause Tooth Discoloration in Prenatal and Neonatal Animals

Tetracycline	Aquari-Cycline Bio-Tet Bovocycline Numerous	14–22 mg/kg PO q 6–8 hr	14–22 mg/kg PO q 6–8 hr	Not common to use in cats because of side effects

Continued

Generic Name	Trade Names	Dog Dose	Cat Dose	Notes
Doxycycline	Vibramycin, Doxirobe gel Numerous	5–10 mg/kg PO q 12–24 hr	5–10 mg/kg PO q 12–24 hr	Good for respiratory infections, brain, CSF, eyes, intracellular, synovial fluid Longer half-life; better central nervous system penetration than tetracycline Periodontal gel available

Oxytetracycline	Oxytet Terramycin Numerous	8–10 mg/kg IM, SC q 24 hr	8–10 mg/kg IM, SC q 24 hr	Give with food if GI upset occurs
Minocycline	Arestin Dynacin Minocin Myrac	5–12 mg/kg PO, IV q 12 hr	6–11 mg/kg PO q 12 hr	
Fluoroquinolones: At High Doses, Bactericidal—Use With Care in Young Patients' Reports Vary With Cartilage Damage. Good for Bone, Intracellular, Prostate, and Synovial Fluid				
Enrofloxacin	Baytril Numerous	5–20 mg/kg PO q 24 hr	2.5–5 mg/kg PO q 24 hr	Use with caution in patients with renal failure

Continued

Generic Name	Trade Names	Dog Dose	Cat Dose	Notes
Orbifloxacin	Orbax	2.5–7.5 mg/kg PO q 24 hr	2.5–7.5 mg/kg PO q 24 hr	
Marbofloxacin	Zeniquin Numerous	2 mg/kg SC once, then 2 mg/kg PO q 24 hr	2.75–5.5 mg/kg PO q 24 hr	Pain and swelling at injection site possible
Lincosamides and Macrolides: Bacteriostatic				
Clindamycin	Antirobe Numerous	5–20 mg/kg IV, SC, PO q 12 hr	11–33 mg/kg PO q 24 hr	Good for bone and prostate Do not administer to rabbits, hamsters, guinea pigs

| Azithromycin | Zithromax AzaSite Zmax | 5–10 mg/kg PO q 12 hr | 7–15 mg/kg PO q 12 hr | Good for intracellular |

Sulfonamides: Bacteriostatic—Can Cause KCS; Good for Brain, CSF, and Prostate

Sulfadiazine and trimethoprim	Tribrissen Di-Trim Numerous	15–30 mg/kg SC, PO q 12 hr	15–30 mg/kg SC, PO q 12 hr	Can precipitate in the kidneys of dehydrated animals
Trimethoprim and sulfame-thoxazole	Bactrim Septra	15–30 mg/kg PO q 12 hr	15–60 mg/kg PO, SC q 24 hr	

Continued

Generic Name	Trade Names	Dog Dose	Cat Dose	Notes
Sulfadimethoxine	Albon Agribon Bactrovet Di-Methox Sulfamed	25–60 mg/kg PO q 24 hr	50–60 mg/kg PO q 24 hr	Coccidiostatic
Miscellaneous				
Metronidazole	Flagyl Numerous	12–25 mg/kg PO q 12 hr	8–25 mg/kg PO q 12 hr	Good for brain, CSF May cause GI upset

ANTIVIRALS

Interferon-α2B	Intron A Pegasys PegIntron Reaferon Sylatron Unitron PEG		5–30 IU **per cat** PO q 24 hr	For the treatment of herpesvirus
Interferon-omega	Virbagen Omega	1–5 million U/kg SC 3 times per week q 4 weeks, then q 1 month	1 million U/kg IV, SC q 24 hr	For the treatment of canine parvovirus, FeLV, and FIV

New and Others

ANTIFUNGALS

Antifungals: Liver Enzyme Elevation Possible; Monitor Liver Effects				
Fluconazole	Diflucan Biocanol Biozolene	5–20 mg/kg PO q 24	5–10 mg/kg PO q 24 hr	Fungistatic is probably most useful for central nervous system infections
Griseofulvin	Fulvicin Grifungal Grisol V	5–10 mg/kg PO q 24 hr	5–10 mg/kg PO q 24 hr	Known teratogen in cats
Itraconazole	Sporanox Itrafungol Itrizole Oriconazole Sporanox	5–10 mg/kg PO q 24 hr	5–10 mg/kg PO q 12 hr	
Ketoconazole	Nizoral Numerous	5–20 mg/kg PO q 12 hr	Avoid in cats	

| Miconazole | Monistat Daktarin
Daktarin
Monistat-Derm | 1%–2%
topically q
4–12 hr | 1%–2%
topically q
24 hr | Used to treat fungal
ophthalmic infections |

New and Others

ANALGESIC AND ANTIINFLAMMATORY AGENTS[62A]

NONSTEROIDAL ANTIINFLAMMATORY DRUGS

Generic Name	Trade Names	Dog Dose	Cat Dose	Notes
Nonsteroidal Antiinflammatory Drugs (NSAIDs): Use With Caution in Liver and Kidney Patients: Avoid in Patients With Gastric Ulcers				
Acetylsalicylic acid	Aspirin Asprisol Compagel Cortaba Dermisol	0–25 mg/kg PO q 12 hr	10–20 mg/kg PO q 48–72 hr	Analgesic, antiinflammatory, and antipyretic

Continued

Generic Name	Trade Names	Dog Dose	Cat Dose	Notes
Carprofen	Rimadyl	4.4 mg/kg PO, SC q 24 hr. Administer approximately 2 hr prior to procedure. Daily dose may be divided and administered q 12 hr		
Deracoxib	Deramaxx Doxidyl Ostimax	1–2 mg/kg PO q 24 hr		Cox 1 sparing: approved for dogs only

Etodolac	EtoGesic, Lodine EtoGesic Lodine Ramodar Ultradol	5–15 mg/kg PO q 24 hr		COX-2 selective; approved for dogs only
Firocoxib	Previcox	5 mg/kg PO q 24 hr		COX-2 selective; approved for dogs only
Ketoprofen	Ketofen, Orudis Numerous	1–2 mg/kg IM, IV, SC q 24 hr	1 mg/kg Po, SQ once	
Meloxicam	Metacam Numerous	0.1–0.2 mg/kg PO, IV, SC q 24 hr	0.3 mg/kg SC once	COX-2 selective; approved for use in cats

Continued

Generic Name	Trade Names	Dog Dose	Cat Dose	Notes
Piroxicam	Feldene	0.3 mg/kg PO q 24 hr	0.13–0.41 mg/kg PO q 24 hr	Can use in cats as an antineoplastic agent
Robenacoxib	Onsior	2 mg/kg PO, SC q 24 hr × maximum of 3 days; first dose should be administered 45 min prior to surgery	1–2.4 mg/kg PO q 24 hr; once clinical response has been observed, dose is adjusted to lowest effective individual dose	Maximum treatment duration of 3 days

New and Others

OTHER ANALGESICS

Generic Name	Trade Name	Dog Dose	Cat Dose	Notes
Grapiprant	Galliprant	2 mg/kg PO q 24 hr		Prostaglandin E_2 EP4 receptor antagonist Less GI and renal side effects than other NSAIDS
Amantadine	Gocovri Lysovir Osmolex ER Symadine Symmetrel Trilasym	3–5 mg/kg PO q 24 hr	2–5 mg/kg PO q 24 hr	

Continued

Generic Name	Trade Name	Dog Dose	Cat Dose	Notes
Gabapentin	Gralise Horizant Neurontin Therapentin	10–30 mg/kg PO q 8 hr	10–40 mg PO q 8 hr	Anticonvulsant
Frunevetmab injection	Solensia		1–2.8 mg/kg SC q month	Monoclonal antibody that blocks pain through inhibition of nerve growth factor
Methocarbamol	Robaxin-V Robaximol Robaxin Robaxin 750	30–60 mg/kg/day PO. Divided into two or three daily doses 44 mg/kg IV to effect	60 mg/kg/day PO. Divided into two or three daily doses 44 mg/kg IV to effect	Skeletal muscle relaxant, may cause sedation

New and Others

CORTICOSTEROIDS

Corticosteroids: Risk of GI Perforations; Use With Caution in Uncontrolled Infections Cushing's and Diabetes Mellitus and Liver Dysfunction

Dexamethasone	Azium, Dexasone Numerous	0.25–1.25 mg **per dog** PO q 24 hr for up to 7 days	0.125–0.5 mg **per cat** IM, IV OR 0.25–0.5 mg **per cat** PO q 24 hr for up to 7 days	Long acting Can induce abortion
Methylprednisolone	Medrol, Depo-Medrol, Solu-Medrol A-Methapred Cortaba	2–40 mg **per dog** IM	10–20 mg **per cat IM**	Intermediate acting

Continued

Triamcinolone	Vetalog Aristocort Azmacort Panolog Kenalog	Induction: 0.22 mg/kg PO SID or 0.1–02 mg/kg IM, SQ Maintenance: 0.055 mg/kg PO SID	0.1–0.2 mg/kg IM, SC	Intermediate acting
Prednisone Prednisolone: required for cats	Meticorten, Deltasone Numerous	Physiologic 0.5 mg/kg PO Antiinflammatory 1.1 mg/kg PO Autoimmune 2.2 mg/kg PO	Physiologic 0.5 mg/kg PO Antiinflammatory 1.1 mg/kg PO Autoimmune 2.2 mg/kg PO	Intermediate acting

Hydrocortisone	A-hydroCort Cortef Cortisporin Forte Topical Kymar Neo-Cortef Solu-Cortef Terra Cortril Vetropolycin HC	10 mg/kg IV q 3–6 hr	10 mg/kg IV q 3–6 hr	Short acting

GLYCOSAMINOGLYCANS

			Nutraceutical
Glucosamine/chondroitin	Many	50–100 mg/kg of glucosamine component PO q 24 hr	27–54 mg/kg of glucosamine component PO q 12 hr × 4–6 weeks, then 13.5–27 mg/kg q 12 hr maintenance
Polysulfated glycosa-minoglycan: PSGAG	Adequan	4.44 mg/kg IM 2 × per week for up to 4 weeks	5 mg/kg SC 2 × weekly for 4 weeks; then q week for 4 weeks; then monthly

OPIOID (NARCOTIC) ANALGESICS

Butorphanol	Torbutrol, Torbugesic, Dolorex Numerous	0.1–0.4 mg/kg SC, IM, IV q 4–6 hr	0.1–0.4 mg/kg SC, IM, IV q 4–6 hr	κ-Agonist/μ-antagonist can be used as a reversal agent for μ-agonist opioids Poor analgesic, good sedative Butorphanol will block effects of full μ-agonists and thus can be used as a partial reversal agent Butorphanol is a DEA Schedule IV drug

Continued

Buprenorphine	Buprenex Simbadol (24 hr formula for cats)	0.01– 0.02 mg/kg q 4–8 hr IM, IV	0.02–0.04 mg/kg q 4–8 hr, IM, IV	Partial μ-agonist Good for moderate-to- severe pain TM administration is unreliable in dogs DEA Schedule III drug
Fentanyl	Duragesic Ionsys	Animal size 2–10 kg cats 10–20 kg 20–30 kg >30 kg CRI 3–6 μg/kg/hr dogs CRI 2–3 μg/kg/hr cats	Fentanyl size patch 25 μg/hr 50 μg/hr 75 μg/hr 100 μg/hr	Continuous, sustained analgesia Agonistic actions at mu opioid DEA Schedule II drug
Hydromorphone	Dilaudid Exalgo Jurnista Palladone	0.05–0.2 mg/ kg q3–4 hr SC, IM	0.05–0.2 mg/kg q3–4 hr SC, IM	μ-Agonist opioid good for severe pain DEA Schedule II drug

Methadone	Dolophine Comfortan Metadol Methadose	0.4–1.0 mg/kg q5–6 hr SC, IM		Full μ-opioid receptor agonist DEA Schedule II drug
Morphine	Infumorph Numerous	0.3–1.0 mg/kg q 2–4 h IM, IV	0.2–0.4 mg/kg q 4–6 h IM, IV	Vomiting usually occurs DEA schedule II drug Agonistic actions at μ-opioid receptors. It is also a κ- and δ-opioid agonist Cautious use with IV administration due to histamine release
Tramadol	Ultram Numerous	4–6 mg/kg q 6–8 hr, IV, IM, PO	2–4 mg/kg q 6–8 h, IV, IM, PO	Weak μ-receptor agonist DEA schedule IV drug Not appropriate as sole analgesic

DERMATOLOGY

Oclacitinib maleate	Apoquel	0.4–0.6 mg/kg PO q 12 hr × 2 weeks, then 0.4–0.6 mg/kg PO q 24 hr	Not for use in dogs <12 months of age May exacerbate neoplastic conditions
Lokivetmab	Cytopoint	2.2–2.3 mg/kg SC q 4–8 weeks prn	
Cyclosporine	Atopica	4–8 mg/kg PO of modified/ microemulsion cyclosporine q 12–24 hr	7 mg/kg PO q 24 hr of modified/micro-emulsion cyclosporine × 4–6 weeks

EAR MEDICATIONS

Ear Medications: Clean Ears Before Instilling Any Medications. Then Do Not Clean During the Treatment

Generic Name	Trade Names	Dog Dose	Cat Dose	Notes
Enrofloxacin and silver sulfadiazine	Baytril Otic	5–15 drops q 12 hr		**Can use with a ruptured tympanic membrane**
Florfenicol, terbinafine, mometasone	Claro	1 dose (1 droperette or 1 mL) per affected ear(s)		DO NOT get in eyes DO NOT use with ruptured tympanic membrane
Florfenicol, terbinafine, betamethasone acetate	Osurnia	1 tube per affected ear Repeat in 7 days	1 tube per affected ear Repeat in 7 days	DO NOT get in eyes DO NOT use if ruptured tympanic membrane

Ear Medications: Clean Ears Before Instilling Any Medications. Then Do Not Clean During the Treatment

Generic Name	Trade Names	Dog Dose	Cat Dose	Notes
Neomycin, dexamethasone, thiabendazole	Tresaderm	5–15 drops q 12 hr	5–15 drops q 12 hr	Also treats ear mites in cats
Silver sulfadiazine	Compound	0.5 mL q 8–12 hr in the ear		Mix 1 part commercial cream with 1–9 parts of water. Rarely can cause hypersensitivity or irritancy. May be good for resistant *Pseudomonas*
Miconazole	Conofite	2–12 drops in affected ear q 12–24 hr	2–12 drops in affected ear q 12–24 hr	Very rarely causes problems with a ruptured tympanic membrane

Gentamicin Gentamicin, mometasone, and clotrimazole Gentamicin, betamethasone, and clotrimazole Gentamicin sulfate and betamethasone valerate Gentamicin and betamethasone	Gentocin Mometamax Otomax Tri-Otic Gentizol Malotic Vet Betagen Otic Genone Otic Gentoved	2–8 drops every 24 hr		DO NOT use with a ruptured tympanic membrane

Continued

Ear Medications: Clean Ears Before Instilling Any Medications. Then Do Not Clean During the Treatment

Generic Name	Trade Names	Dog Dose	Cat Dose	Notes
Neomycin, thiostrepton, triamcinolone, nystatin Nystatin, neomycin sulfate, triamcinolone acetonide Neomycin sulfate, isoflupredone acetate, tetracaine hydrochloride	Panolog Animax Derma-Vet Entederm Dermalone Restorin Neo-Predef Tritop	3–5 drops TID	3–5 drops TID	Hearing loss is possible DO NOT use if tympanic membrane ruptured

Ivermectin	Acarexx	0.5 mL per ear	0.5 mL 0.01% tube (Acarexx) topically into each external ear canal	Ear mites
Milbemycin oxime	Milbemite		0.25 mL (4% soln) topically into each external ear canal	Ear mites
Pyrethrin, technical piperonyl butoxide, dicarboximide, Di-n-P isoinchomeronate	Otomite Plus Mita-Clear	1 drop per pound body weight	2 drops per pound body weight	Ear mites

EYE MEDICATIONS

Generic Name	Trade Names	Dog Dose	Cat Dose	Notes
Atropine	None	1 drop of 1% atropine in affected eye(s) q 6–24 hr		Dilates the eye Can be used to help with pain Do NOT use with glaucoma
Cyclosporine	Optimmune Cequa Restasis	Apply 1/4-in. or 1/2-cm strip of ointment to affected eye(s) q 12 hr		Treat KCS Do not use with viral or fungal infections
Dexamethasone 1%	Maxidex Maxitrol Tobradex	1–2 drops in affected eye(s) q 1–6 hr depending on severity of disease		

Diclofenac	Voltaren	1 drop of 0.1% solution q 6–12 hr	Should be used with discretion in patients prone to secondary glaucoma Used for anterior uveitis
Dorzolamide	Trusopt	1 drop OU q 6–8 hr.	Used to treat glaucoma
Tobramycin	AKTob Tobradex Tobrasone Tobrex Zylet	0.5-in. ribbon of 0.3% tobramycin ointment in affected eye(s) q 8–12 hr 1–2 drops of 0.3% tobramycin solution in affected eye(s) q 4 hr	Antibiotics
Neopolybac		Apply 1/4-in. ribbon TID Apply 1–2 drops TID	Can cause allergic reaction in cats

Continued

Generic Name	Trade Names	Dog Dose	Cat Dose	Notes
Neopolydex		Apply 1/4-in. ribbon TID Apply 1–2 drops TID		DO NOT use with corneal ulcers Can cause allergic reaction in cats
Tropicamide	Mydriacyl Mydriafair Paremyd Tropicacyl	1 drop of 1% tropicamide per eye		Dilates the eye
Latanoprost	Numerous	1 drop of 0.005% solution per affected eye q 10–15min × 2–3 doses Maintenance 1 drop of 0.005% solution per affected eye q 24hr		Glaucoma treatment

Serum	None	Pull blood spin down and remove the serum. Administer 2 drops q 2–8 hr	Good for 2 weeks if kept in refrigerator Treatment of cornea ulcers
Lubricants	i-drop vet gel Optixcare Artificial Tears	1 drop prn	Anesthesia KCS
Cidofovir	Empovir Vistide		1 drop of 0.5% cidofovir in 1% carboxy-methylcellulose OU q 12hr	Viral ocular disease

Continued

Generic Name	Trade Names	Dog Dose	Cat Dose	Notes
Proparacaine	Ak-Taine Alcaine Ophthaine Ophthetic	3–5 administrations of 1–2 drops to cornea		Local anesthetic
Ofloxacin	Ocuflox	1–2 drops into affected eye(s) q 30 min during waking hours and q 4–6 hr at night × 2 days, then 1–2 drops q 1 hr during waking hours × 5–7 days, then 1–2 drops q 6 hr × 2 days		

ANTICONVULSANTS

Generic Name	Trade Names	Dog Dose	Cat Dose	Notes
Phenobarbital	Luminal Numerous	1–3 mg/kg PO q 12 hr Status epilepticus 16–20 mg/kg IV once		Usually first choice for idiopathic epilepsy Check therapeutic range after 2 weeks Monitor the liver Slow elevation of ALP is not cause for alarm
Potassium bromide (KBr)	Numerous	25–68 mg/kg PO q 24 hr; dosage can be divided and should be adjusted to clinical response		Used as an adjunct in management of idiopathic epilepsy

Continued

Generic Name	Trade Names	Dog Dose	Cat Dose	Notes
Diazepam	Valium Diastat Diazemuls Diazepam Intensol	0.5 mg/kg per rectum	1.25–2.5 mg **per cat** per rectum q 2 hr	Used to control status epilepticus
Zonisamide	Exceglan Excegram Excegran Tremode Trerief Zonegran	5–10 mg/kg PO q 12 hr	5–10 mg/kg/day PO q 24 hr	Can be used for seizures as a primary or adjunct agent
Levetiracetam	Keppra Apo-levetiracetam Kepcet tablets Kerron tablets	7–25 mg/kg PO q 8 hr	20 mg/kg PO q 8 hr	Can be used for seizures as a primary or adjunct agent

CARDIOVASCULAR DRUGS

Generic Name	Trade Names	Dog Dose	Cat Dose	Notes
Pimobendan	Vetmedin Acardi Cardisure Pimocard Pimotab	0.5 mg/kg PO; divided into 2 administrations q 12 hr using suitable combination of whole and half tablets	0.25–0.3 mg/kg PO q 12 hr	Used to manage congestive heart failure Inotropic Contraindicated in cases of hypertrophic cardiomyopathy, aortic stenosis
Benazepril	Lotensin Fortekor	0.25–0.5 mg/kg PO q 12–24 hr	0.25–0.5 mg/kg PO q 24 hr	For adjunctive treatment of heart failure ACE inhibitor

Continued

Generic Name	Trade Names	Dog Dose	Cat Dose	Notes
Enalapril	Enacard, Vasotec	0.5–1 mg/kg PO q 12–24 hr	0.25–0.5 mg/kg PO q 12 hr	ACE inhibitor
Furosemide	Lasix, Disal, Diuride, Salix	1–4 mg/kg PO, IM, SC q 8–24 hr 2–8 mg/kg IV	0.5–2.5 mg/kg PO, IM, IV q 8–24 hr	Caution in dehydrated patientsDiuretic
Spironolactone	Aldactone Aldactazide Cardalis Prilactone Tempora	2 mg/kg PO q 24 hr	1.7–3.3 mg/kg PO q 24 hr	Potassium-sparing diuretic

ANTIARRHYTHMICS

Generic Name	Trade Names	Dog Dose	Cat Dose	Notes
Lidocaine	Xylocaine Dermacool Ekyflogyl	2–3 mg/kg IV bolus over 5 sec. Total dosage not to exceed 8 mg/kg. Repeat in 2–3 min if first dose unsuccessful; final dose after 2–3 min prn. Use cautiously with patients with concurrent atrioventricular block[22]		Do not use lidocaine with epinephrine preparations for intravenous solutions Antiarrhythmic-supraventricular tachycardia

Continued

Generic Name	Trade Names	Dog Dose	Cat Dose	Notes
Procainamide	Pronestyl, Procan Procanbid	Chronic maintenance 20–40 mg/kg PO q 6–8 hr for prompt release procainamide 2–4 mg/kg slow IV bolus. Do not exceed total dosage of 20 mg/kg; ±follow with 20–50 mcg/kg/min IV CRI or 7–10 mg/kg IM q 6–8 hr		Supraventricular tachycardia Chronic management of ventricular premature contractions and ventricular tachycardia
Quinidine	Quinidex	6–11 mg/kg IM q 6 hr; some dogs convert from atrial fibrillation to a sinus rhythm within 24 hr of therapy 6–16 mg/kg PO q 8 hr	Use with caution with other antiarrhythmics	Atrial fibrillation in dogs without heart disease Ventricular arrhythmias

RESPIRATORY DRUGS[62]

Generic Name	Trade Names	Dog Dose	Cat Dose	Notes
Bronchodilators				
Albuterol	Ventolin, Proventil	1–4 **mg per dog** PO q 12 hr	108 mcg **per cat** via inhalation/ metered spray q 30–60 min until respiratory distress resolves, then 108 mcg per cat as needed	Most adverse effec s are dose related and generally transient
Terbutaline	Brethine	1.0–5.0 mg/dog PO SID-TID	0.625–1.25 mg per cat PO BID EMERGENCY 0.01 mg/kg IV, SC, IM	

Continued

Generic Name	Trade Names	Dog Dose	Cat Dose	Notes
Aminophylline	Many	11 mg/kg PO TID	5 mg/kg PO BID	Do not inject air into multidose vials; CO_2 causes drug to precipitate; narrow therapeutic index Weak affect in cats
Theophylline		10 mg/kg PO BID. Start with 1/2 dose for 3–4 days and if well tolerated, increase to full dose	20 mg/kg SID in the evening	Available in sustained-release oral dose form
Antihistamines				
Cyproheptadine	Periactin		2 mg PO SID–BID prn	Also used for appetite stimulation in cats

Diphenhy-dramine	Benadryl	2–4 mg/kg IM, PO, SC q 8–12 hr	2–4 mg/kg PO q 6–8 hr	IV form used to counteract anaphylactic reactions
Trimeprazine (with prednisolone)	Temaril-P	Weight of dog initial dosage Up to 10 lb 1/2 tablet, twice daily 11–20 lb 1 tablet, twice daily 21–40 lb 2 tablets, twice daily Over 40 lb 3 tablets, twice daily		Combination antihistamine and corticosteroid

Continued

Generic Name	Trade Names	Dog Dose	Cat Dose	Notes
Antitussives				
Butorphanol	Torbutrol, Torbugesic	0.05–0.12 mg/kg PO BID–TID		Narcotic cough suppressant
Hydrocodone	Hycodan, Tussigon	0.22 mg/kg PO BID–QID		Narcotic cough suppressant
Dextrometho-phan	Robitussin	1–2 mg/kg PO TID–QID		Nonnarcotic cough suppressant; available over the counter
Mucolytics				
Acetylcysteine	Mucomyst	IV, PO, inhalation		Antidote for acetaminophen toxicity

GASTROINTESTINAL DRUGS[62]

Generic Name	Trade Names	Dog Dose	Cat Dose	Notes
Antiemetics: Do Not Use If Gastrointestinal Obstruction				
Maropitant citrate	Cerenia	1 mg/kg SC q 24hr for up to 5 d 2 mg/kg PO × 24 hr	1 mg/kg SC or IV over 1–2 min q 24 hr for up to 5 days 4 mg **per cat** PO q 24 hr	
Dimenhydrinate	Dramamine	4–8 mg/kg IM, IV, PO q 8 hr	4–8 mg/kg PO q 8 hr	Used primarily for motion sickness Dilute and give slowly if using IV
Meclizine	Antivert	4–8 mg/kg PO q 8 hr	1–2 mg/kg PO q 24 hr	Primarily used for motion sickness

Continued

Generic Name	Trade Names	Dog Dose	Cat Dose	Notes
Metoclopramide	Reglan Emeprid Metomide Vomend	0.2–0.5 mg/kg IM, IV, PO, SC	0.2–0.5 mg/kg IM, IV, PO, SC	Promotility agent; inhibits gastroesophageal reflux
Ondansetron	Zofran	0.1–1 mg/kg IV, PO q 6–12 hr	0.5–1.0 mg/kg PO, IV q 6–12 hr	
Antiulcer				
Cimetidine	Tagamet	2.5–10 mg/kg IV, PO, SC q 6–12 hr		Oral form available over the counter; do not refrigerate injectable form
Famotidine	Pepcid	0.1–0.2 mg/kg IM, IV, PO, SC q 12 hr	0.2–1 mg/kg IV, PO, SC q 12–24 hr	Oral form available over the counter

| Sucralfate | Carafate | 0.5–1 g **per dog** PO q 8 hr | Forms a protective barrier at gastric ulcer site; administer 60 min before other medications or food |
| Omeprazole | Prilosec | 0.5–1 mg/kg PO q 24 hr | A proton-pump inhibitor, may affect absorption rates of drugs requiring a low stomach pH; do not split caplets |

Continued

Generic Name	Trade Names	Dog Dose	Cat Dose	Notes
Appetite Stimulants				
Diazepam	Valium		0.05 mg/kg IV	Effective immediately Much smaller dose than for sedation
Capromorelin	Entyce Elura	3 mg/kg PO q 24 hr	1–3 mg/kg PO q 24 hr	
Mirtazapine	Mirataz Avanza Axit Remeron Zispin	0.5–1.5 mg/kg PO q 24 hr, not to exceed 30 mg/dog/day	1.88 **mg per cat** q 12–24 hr to 3.5 mg/ cat PO q 72 hr	
Laxatives				
Magnesium salts	Milk of Magnesia	5–50 mL **per dog** PO q 4–6 hr, using 80 mg/mL	5–10 mL **per cat** PO q 4–6 hr, using 80 mg/mL	Hyperosmotic; holds water in gastrointestinal tract and softens stool

Bisacodyl	Dulcolax	5–15 mg per **medium- to large-sized dog**	5 mg PO q 24 hr	Stimulant laxative
Lactulose	Enulose	0.22 mL/kg PO q 8 hr	0.22 mL/kg PO q 8 hr	Hyperosmotic; also used to reduce blood ammonia levels in hepatic disease
Docusate	Colace, DSS	50–200 mg **per dog** PO q 24h 250 mg **per dog** per rectum. Repeat in 1 hr if necessary	50 mg **per cat** PO q 24 hr 250 mg **per cat** per rectum. Repeat in 1 hr if necessary	Stool softener; watch hydration status

Continued

Generic Name	Trade Names	Dog Dose	Cat Dose	Notes
Antidiarrheals				
Diphenoxylate/atropine	Lomotil	0.1–0.2 mg/kg PO q 12 hr	0.05–0.1 mg/kg PO q 12 hr	Opiates reduce gut motility; small amount of atropine reduces other narcotic effects
Kaolin/pectin	K-P-Sol	110 mg/kg PO kaolin (1 tablet per 9 kg) q 8 hr in combination with 5.6 mg/kg pectin and 0.07 billion cfu/kg *Enterococcus faecium*; tablets may be administered whole or crumbled and given with meal		
Bismuth subsalicylate	Pepto-Bismol Kaopectate	4.4–8.8 mg/kg PO q 6 hr × 36 hr, then q 12 hr × 2–3 days	8.75–17.5 mg/kg PO q 12 hr × 3 days	May discolor the stool to black

Emetics

Apomorphine	Numerous	0.25 mg/kg PO or ocular once 0.05 mg/kg IV 0.1 mg/kg SC	If vomiting does not occur with initial dose, subsequent doses are not likely to be effective and may induce toxicity; wear gloves when handling
Ropinirole	Clevor Requip	**Body weight in kilograms** / **Total number of eye drops** 1.8–5 / 1 5.1–10 / 2 10.1–20 / 3 20.1–35 / 4 35.1–60 / 6 60.1–100 / 8	

Continued

Generic Name	Trade Names	Dog Dose	Cat Dose	Notes
Miscellaneous				
Ursodiol	Actigall Urso	10–15 mg/kg PO q 24 hr with food		Use to increase the flow of bile
SAMe	Denosyl Denamarin Novifit S Zentonil	20 mg/kg PO q 24 hr		Nutraceutical agent used as an adjunct to treatment of liver disease
Pancreatic supplement	Viokase PANCREZYME Powder	Feed as directed to label		Products contain lipase, amylase, protease enzymes; cats strongly dislike the taste of powder forms
New and Others				

ENDOCRINE DRUGS[62]

Generic Name	Trade Names	Routes	Dose	Notes
Estrogen-Responsive Urinary Incontinence				
Diethylstil-bestrol (DES)	Agostilben Apstil Distilbène Honvol Stilboestrol Stilboestrol	0.1 mg/kg PO q 24 h × 3–5 d, then up to 1 mg **per dog** weekly	0.5 mg **per cat** PO q 24 hr × 2 weeks	Used to treat estrogen-responsive urinary incontinence; toxic to bone marrow; contraindicated in pregnancy
Phenylpropano-lamine	Proin Continence Dexatrim Propalin Urilin	1–2 mg/kg PO q 8–24 hr	1.5–2.2 mg/kg PO q 8–12 hr	Treat urinary incontinence

Continued

Generic Name	Trade Names	Routes	Dose	Notes
Progestins				
Megestrol	Ovaban, Megace	0.45 mg/kg/day PO × 8 days		For false pregnancy; contraindicated in pregnancy; can induce hypoadrenocorticism, personality changes, transient diabetes, and has many other side effects
Pituitary Hormones				
Oxytocin	Pitocin	2.5–10 IU **per dog** IM, IV, SC	2.5–10 IU **per cat** IM, IV, SC	Induction and enhancement of uterine contractions at parturition Ensure fetal obstruction not present

Corticotropin	Cortrosyn	5 mcg/kg IV or IM	125 mcg per cat IV or IM	ACTH stimulation test draw preblood sample Administer corticotropin Draw post-blood sample 1 hr later

Hypoadrenocorticism (Addison's Disease) Treatments

Fludrocortisone	Florinef	0.1–0.5 mg **per dog** PO q 12 hr	0.1–0.2 mg **per cat** PO divided q 12 hr	Mineralocorticoid
Desoxycorticosterone (DOCP)	Percorten-V	1.5–2.2 mg/kg IM q 25 days	12.5 mg IM q 3–4 weeks	Mineralocorticoid

Continued

Hyperadrenocorticism (Cushing's Disease) Treatment

Generic Name	Trade Names	Routes	Dose	Notes
Trilostane	Vetoryl	2.2–6.7 mg/kg PO q 24hr	3.3 mg/kg PO q 12hr, adjust dose, interval as needed	Recheck ACTH stim in 2 weeks
Selegiline (l-deprenyl)	Anipryl, Eldepryl	1 mg/kg PO q 24hr; preferably in morning; if no improvement after 2 months, increase dosage to maximum of 2 mg/kg q 24hr and monitor closely for adverse effects; reevaluate if no improvement after 1 month or if clinical signs progress		For the treatment of hyperadrenocorticism; also used in the treatment of canine cognitive dysfunction

Mitotane	Lysodren		INDUCTION: 40–50 mg/kg/day PO × 7–10 days MAINTENANCE: 50 mg/kg PO weekly in 2–3 divided doses	
Antidiabetics				
Regular insulin	Humulin R	2.2 IU/kg/day IV CRI	1.1–2.2 IU/kg/day IV CRI	Diabetic ketoacidosis
Intermediate acting	Vetsulin Humulin N Novolin N	0.25–0.5 U/kg SC q 12 hr		U-40 for Vetsulin U-100 for Humulin N or Novolin N. Use matching syringe Should be shaken vigorously Keep refrigerated Does not always work well in cats

Continued

Generic Name	Trade Names	Routes	Dose	Notes
Glargine insulin	Lantus		0.25–0.5 U/kg SC, q 12 h	U-100: Use matching syringe Roll insulin do not shake Keep refrigerated
Glipizide	Glucotrol		2.5–5 mg **per cat** PO q 12hr; administer with food	Oral hypoglycemic agents
Hypothyroidism Treatment				
Levothyroxine	Soloxine, Thyrozine Numerous	0.022 mg/kg PO q 12 hr	0.02–0.04 mg/kg PO q 24 hr or divided q 12 hr	

Hyperthyroidism Treatment

Methimazole	Felimazole Tapazole		2.5–5 mg **per cat** PO q 8–12 hr	Can absorb through skin best to use coated capsules

ANTIDOTES

Generic Name	Trade Names	Dog Dose	Cat Dose	Uses and Indications
Acetylcysteine	Mucomyst	140 mg/kg IV, PO then 70 mg/kg IV, PO q 6 hr × 5–7 treatments	140 mg/kg IV, PO then 70 mg/kg IV, PO q 6 hr × 5–7 treatments	Acetaminophen toxicity
Atropine	Many	0.2 mg/kg, administer 1/4 of dose IV and remainder IM or SC	0.2 mg/kg, administer 1/4 of dose IV and remainder IM or SC	Organophosphate toxicity

Continued

Generic Name	Trade Names	Dog Dose	Cat Dose	Uses and Indications
Calcium EDTA	Calcium Disodium Versenate	100 mg/kg SC q 24 hr × 2–5 days. Divide daily dose into four portions; dilute to final concentration of 10 mg calcium EDTA per mL of 5% dextrose and deliver at different SC sites; do not exceed 2 g per dog per day; rest 5 days and repeat as necessary	5 mg/kg IV slowly in divided daily doses	Lead poisoning

| Fomepizole (4-MP) | Antizol Antizol-Vet Fomepizole | 20 mg/kg IV followed by 15 mg/kg IV at 12 hr and 24 hr, then 5 mg/kg IV at 36 hr. If signs have not improved or ethylene glycol test is still positive, continue with 5 mg/kg IV q 12 hr | 125 mg/kg IV followed by 31.25 mg/kg IV at 12 hr, 24 hr, and 36 hr. This regimen was successful only if initiated within 3 hr of exposure to lethal dose of ethylene glycol | Ethylene glycol toxicity |

Continued

Generic Name	Trade Names	Dog Dose	Cat Dose	Uses and Indications
Activated charcoal	Actidose Adsorba CharcoAid D-Tox-Besc EZ-Char Insta-Char Liqua-Char ToxiBan UAA Gel	1–4 g/kg PO as aqueous slurry (~1 g per 5 mL water). May be repeated at 4–6 hr intervals		

EUTHANASIA DRUGS

Generic Name	Trade Names	Dog Dose	Cat Dose	Uses and Indications
Pentobarbital Pentobarbital with phenytoin	Euthansol Euthasol Fatal-Plus Beuthanasia-D	108 mg/kg (1 mL/5kg) IC, IP, IV (IV preferred)		IV (slow to effect) Class II–controlled substance

SURGERY AND ANESTHESIA

NORMAL HEART RATE AND BLOOD PRESSURE
IN DOGS AND CATS[21]

ETCO$_2$	SPO$_2$	Temperature	Heart Rate	Respiration	Normal Blood Pressure (mm Hg)				
					Systolic	Diastolic	Mean (Awake)	Mean (Anesthesia)	
Dogs									
35–45 mm Hg	95%–99%	101–102.5	80–140	8–20	90–160	50–90	85–120	70–99	
Cats									
35–45 mm Hg	95%–99%	100.4–102.5	140–200	8–30	90–160	50–90	85–120	70–99	

ETCO$_2$, End-tidal carbon dioxide level; *MAP*, mean arterial pressure; *SaO$_2$*, arterial oxygen saturation.

NORMAL BLOOD GAS VALUES[7,a]

Sample	pH	PCO_2 (mm Hg)	HCO_3 (mm Hg)	PO_2 (mm Hg)
Dog venous	7.32–7.40	33–50	18–26	
Dog arterial	7.36–7.44	36–44	18–26	85–100
Cat venous	7.28–7.41	33–45	18–23	
Cat arterial	7.36–7.44	28–32	17–22	85–100

[a]In-house normal values should be established if the machine does not come with a published reference range.

ANESTHESIA MACHINES[29]

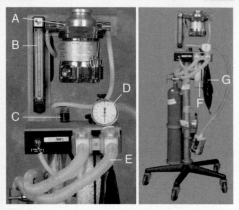

Standard anesthetic machine. Individual components are identified. *A*, Vaporizer; *B*, flowmeter; *C*, oxygen flush valve; *D*, pressure manometer; *E*, circle breathing circuit; *F*, soda lime canister; *G*, rebreathing bag.

BREATHING CIRCUITS

NONREBREATHING CIRCUITS[3,59]

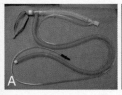
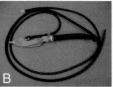

For patients weighing less than 7 kg. (A) Modified Jackson Rees nonrebreathing circuit. (B) Modified Mapleson D nonrebreathing circuit.

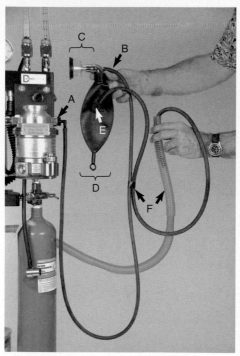

Parts of a nonrebreathing circuit. *A*, Outlet port of the vaporizer with keyed fitting; *B*, fresh gas inlet; *C*, connector with mask attached; *D*, reservoir bag; *E*, pressure relief valve; *F*, scavenging hose.

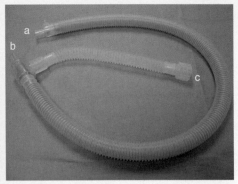

For patients weighing more than 7 kg. Universal F rebreathing circuit (a) connects to the endotracheal tube; (b) connects to the inspiratory valve; (c) connects to the expiratory valve.

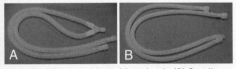

(A) Large-diameter rebreathing circuit. (B) Small-diameter rebreathing circuit.

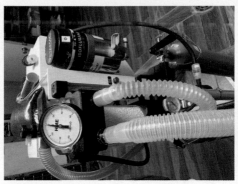

Proper connection of a rebreathing system.

REBREATHING BAG SIZES[11]

Rebreathing Bag Sizes: 5 × tidal volume = bag size in milliliters (mL). Tidal volume calculated as 10–20 mL/kg of body weight.	
Up to 3 kg	500 mL
4–7 kg	1 L
8–15 kg	2 L
16–50 kg	3 L
51–150 kg	5 L
Over 150 kg	30 L

OXYGEN FLOW RATE VALUES[11,61]

OXYGEN FLOW RATE QUICK LOOK-UP CHART FOR REBREATHING SYSTEMS[11,61]

Weight (kg)	Closed System[a] (5–10 mL/kg/min, SA)	Guideline Oxygen Flows (L/min)		
		Semiclosed During Maintenance (20–40 mL/kg/min, SA)	Semiclosed During Induction, Recovery, and Changes (50–100 mL/kg/min, SA)	Semiclosed With Minimal Rebreathing[b] (200–300 mL/kg/min)
2.5	0.1	0.25	0.25–0.3	0.5–0.8
5	0.1	0.25	0.3–0.5	1–1.5
10	0.1	0.25–0.4	0.5–1	2–3
15	0.1–0.15	0.3–0.6	0.8–1.5	3–4.5
20	0.1–0.2	0.4–0.8	1–2	4–5
25	0.13–0.25	0.5–1	1.3–2.5	5

30	0.15–0.3	0.6–1.2	1.5–3	5
40	0.2–0.4	0.8–1.6	2–4	5
50	0.25–0.5	1–2	2.5–5	5
60	0.3–0.6	1.2–2.4	3–5	5
70	0.35–0.7	1.4–2.8	3.5–5	5
80	0.4–0.8	1.6–3.2	4–5	5
90	0.45–0.9	1.8–3.6	4.5–5	5
100	0.5–1	2–4	5	5
150	0.75–1.5	3–5	5	5

[a]At flow rates less than 250 mL/min, vaporizer output may not be accurate.
[b]Minimal rebreathing occurs only when the oxygen flow is greater than or equal to the RMV.

OXYGEN FLOW RATE QUICK LOOK-UP CHART FOR NONREBREATHING SYSTEMS[11,61]

Wt. (kg)	Guideline Oxygen Flows (L/min)	
	Mapleson A (Magill)[a] Modified Mapleson A (Lack)[a] Modified Mapleson D (Bain Coaxial)[b] (0.75–1.0 × RMV)	Modified Mapleson D (Bain Coaxial with No Rebreathing) Mapleson E (Ayre's T-piece) Mapleson F (Norman Mask Elbow and Jackson-Rees) (2–3 × RMV)
1–2.5	0.25–0.5	0.5–1.5
2.5–5	0.5–1	1.5–2.5
5–7	1–1.5	2–3

[a]Controlled ventilation is not recommended with these systems.

[b]Flows listed in this column are believed to result in minimal rebreathing with this system during spontaneous ventilation.

A, Hose connector; *B*, body; *C*, cuff indicator; *D*, cuff; *E*, Murphy eye.

PREANESTHETICS, SEDATIVES, ANESTHETICS

PREANESTHETICS, SEDATIVES, ANESTHETICS[62A]

Generic Name	Trade Names	Dog Dose	Cat Dose	Notes
Barbiturates				
Thiopental	Pentothal	8–22 mg/kg IV to effect	8–22 mg/kg IV to effect	May adsorb to plastic IV bags and lines; ultra–short acting
Tranquilizers and Sedatives				
Acepromazine	PromAce, Atravet	0.55–1.1 mg/kg IM, IV, SC	1.1–2.2 mg/kg IM, IV, SC	Most clinicians use much lower doses. Do not use in conjunction with organophosphates; may cause paradoxical central nervous system stimulation, hypotension

Dexmedetomidine	Dexdomitor	2–20 mcg/kg IM, IV	20–40 mcg/kg IM, IV	Alpha-2 agonist often used as CRI (see below)
Diazepam, midazolam	Valium, Versed	0.1–0.4 mg/kg IM/SC/IV	0.1–0.4 mg/kg IM/SC/IV	Used as anxiolytic, muscle relaxant, appetite stimulant, perianesthetic, and anticonvulsant
Medetomidine	Domitor	750 mcg/m² IV 1000 mcg/m² IM	10–40 mcg/kg IV 40–80 mcg/kg IM	Alpha-2 agonist used for sedation or analgesia in young, healthy animals; adverse effects, such as bradycard a, can be treated by reversing the drug

Continued

Generic Name	Trade Names	Dog Dose	Cat Dose	Notes
Xylazine	Rompun, Anased	1.1 mg/kg IV 2.2 mg/kg IM	1.1 mg/kg IV 2.2 mg/kg IM	Alpha-2 agonist used for sedation analgesia in young, healthy animals; available in 20 and 100 mg/mL; check concentration before administering; respiratory depression and vomiting are common side effects and can be treated by reversing the drug
Miscellaneous Anesthetics				
Ketamine	Ketaset, Vetalar	10 mg/kg IM 10 min following 1.3–2 mg/kg xylazine (dogs >25 kg use lower dosage) and atropine	11–33 mg/ kg IM	Dissociative anesthetic; most reflexes and muscle tone are maintained; no somatic analgesia exists

Propofol	Rapinovet, PropoFlo, Diprivan	5–7 mg/kg IV	8.0–13.2 mg/kg IV	Rapid induction and recovery; drug is carried in an egg lecithin and soy base, which supports bacterial growth
Tiletamine/zolazepam	Telazol	2.2–4.4 mg/kg IV	10.6–12.5 mg/kg IM	Tiletamine is a dissociative anesthetic; zolazepam is a tranquilizer; most reflexes are retained
Etomidate	Amidate	0.5–4 mg/kg IV	0.5–4 mg/kg IV	Minimal effects on the cardiovascular and respiratory system occur; given alone causes myoclonus

Continued

Generic Name	Trade Names	Dog Dose	Cat Dose	Notes
Guaifenesin	Guailaxin	2.2 mL/kg/hr IV using 5% dextrose in water containing 50 mg/mL guaifenesin, 0.25 mg/mL xylazine, and 1 mg/mL ketamine	Not used	Muscle relaxant perianesthetic when given parenterally; expectorant when given orally
Alfaxalone	Alfaxan	1–15 mg/kg IV, IM	0.5–5 mg/kg IV, IM	Rapid metabolism, little cumulative effect; discard unused contents within 6 hr of opening vial
Anticholinergics				
Atropine	Many	0.02–0.04 mg/kg IV, IM	0.02–0.04 mg/kg IV, IM	Used for cardiac support

Glycopyrrolate	Robinul-V	0.011 mg/kg IM, IV, SC	0.011 mg/kg IM	Used for cardiac support; not suitable for emergency use
Reversal Agents				
Naloxone	Narcan	0.002–0.02 mg/kg IV, IM	0.002–0.02 mg/kg IV, IM	Reverse effects of narcotics
Yohimbine	Yobine	0.11 mg/kg IV slowly	0.1 mg/kg IV, IM	Reversal of xylazine (Rompun)
Atipamezole	Antisedan	3.75 mg/m² IM.	3.75 mg/m² IM.	Formulated so that volume for injection is the same (mL for mL) as the recommended dose of medetomidine or dexmedetomidine

MLK CANINE OR FELINE PATIENT WEIGHT IN KILOGRAMS[86-88,98,99]

Propofol[a]	Concentration	Loading Dose[b]	CRI	
	10 mg/mL injection (PropoFlo, PropoFlo 28, Rapinovet)	4–6 mg/kg IV slow	Created with nondiluted propofol for IV delivery ranges	
			Sedation	0.1–0.3 mg/kg/min
			Anesthesia	0.4–0.6 mg/kg/min

[a]Notes: Sedation dose can be helpful as adjunct agent for difficult anesthetic cases or for tracheostomy cases. Anesthesia dose can be used as TIVA for MRI, vent cases, refractory seizures, or surgery (with the addition of analgesia). Avoid repeated dosing in felines (may contribute to Heinz body anemia).

[b]For anesthetic induction; if patient is already anesthetized, this may not be necessary.

PROPOFOL CRI: CANINE OR FELINE PATIENT WEIGHT IN KILOGRAMS[86–88,98,99]

Propofol CRI in mL/hr	5	10	15	20	25	30	35	40	45	50
Sedation	3–9	6–18	9–27	12–24	15–36	18–54	21–63	24–72	27–81	30–9
Anesthesia	12–18	24–36	36–54	48–72	60–90	72–108	84–126	96–144	108–162	120–180

Canine or Feline Patient Weight in Kilograms

Propofol CRI in mL/min	5	10	15	20	25	30	35	40	45	50
Sedation	0.05–0.15	0.10–0.3	0.15–0.45	0.2–0.6	0.25–0.60	0.30–0.9	0.35–1.05	0.40–1.20	0.45–1.35	0.50–1.50
Anesthesia	0.2–0.3	0.4–0.6	0.6–0.9	0.8–1.2	1.0–1.5	1.2–1.8	1.4–2.10	1.6–2.40	1.8–2.70	2.0–3.0

CAPNOGRAPHY

COMMON CHANGES IN THE CAPNOGRAM AND ASSOCIATED CAUSES[61]

Changes	Causes	Capnogram Readout
No waveform	Esophageal intubation Machine malfunction Sensor not properly connected	40 —————— 0 ——————
Sudden loss of waveform	Apnea Cardiac arrest ET tube disconnected Accidental extubation Complete ET tube–circuit obstruction Machine malfunction Ventilator malfunction (if using one)	40 0
Gradual decrease in ETCO$_2$	Hypothermia Hyperventilation	40 0

Rapid decrease in ETCO$_2$	Cardiac arrest Severe blood loss Pulmonary embolism Sudden hypotension	
Gradual increase in ETCO$_2$	Hypoventilation Malignant hyperthermia Fever Muscle tremors, shivering	
Rapid increase in ETCO$_2$	Return of spontaneous circulation after successful CPCR	
Increase in baseline CO$_2$ (usually with a gradual increase in ETCO$_2$)	Malfunction of expiratory unidirectional valve Saturation of CO$_2$ absorbent Contamination of sensor with secretions	

Continued

Changes	Causes	Capnogram Readout
Sudden, temporary increase in ETCO$_2$	Release of a tourniquet Administration of sodium bicarbonate	
Increased angle of the plateau	Asthma or other obstructive lung diseases	
Slow upward stroke	Asthma or other obstructive lung diseases Obstructed breathing circuit	
Sloppy upstroke and downstroke	Leaky cuff Partially kinked endotracheal tube	

CPCR, Cardiopulmonary-cerebral resuscitation.

ELECTRODE PLACEMENT FOR STANDARD LIMB LEADS (I, II, III, AVR, AVL, AVF)[15]

RA, white	Right forelimb; clip to skin just proximal to the olecranon (caudal triceps region)
LA, black	Left forelimb; clip to skin just proximal to the olecranon (caudal triceps region)
RL, green	Right hind limb; clip to skin just proximal to the stifle (cranial thigh); ground wire
LL, red	Left hind limb; clip to skin just proximal to the stifle (cranial thigh)

AVl, augmented vector left; *AVF,* augmented vector foot; *AVR,* augmented vector right; *LA,* left arm; *LL,* left leg; *RA,* right arm; *RL,* right leg.

NORMAL CANINE P-QRS-T COMPLEX[19]

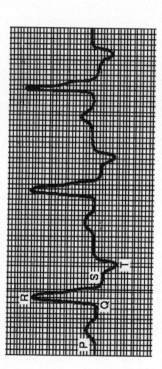

Normal lead II electrocardiographic complex. Atrial depolarization is indicated by the P wave. Following the P wave, there is a short delay in the A–V node (P–R segment), after which the ventricles depolarize and produce the QRS complex. This S–T segment and the T wave represent ventricular repolarization.

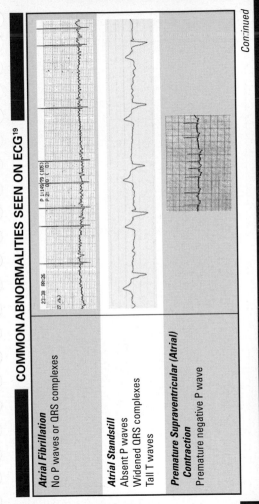

COMMON ABNORMALITIES SEEN ON ECG[19]

Atrial Fibrillation
No P waves or QRS complexes

Atrial Standstill
Absent P waves
Widened QRS complexes
Tall T waves

Premature Supraventricular (Atrial) Contraction
Premature negative P wave

Continued

349

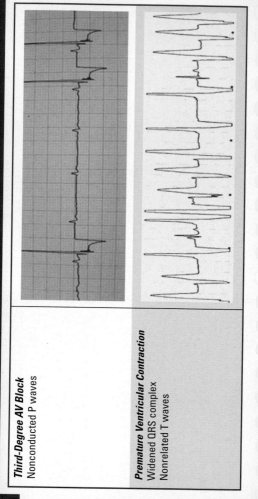

Third-Degree AV Block
Nonconducted P waves

Premature Ventricular Contraction
Widened QRS complex
Nonrelated T waves

SURGICAL INSTRUMENTS[44,59]

HEMOSTATIC FORCEPS[44]

Photo	Name	Construction and Functional Description	Nickname
	Halsted	Serrations are full horizontal Straight and curved Length 5" (12.7 cm)	Mosquito Clamp

Continued

Photo	Name	Construction and Functional Description	Nickname
	Hartman	Serrations are full horizontal Straight and curved Length 3½″ (8.9 cm)	Mosquito Clamp/ Baby Mosquito

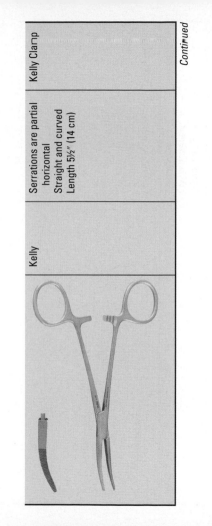

| | Kelly | Serrations are partial horizontal
Straight and curved
Length 5½″ (14 cm) | Kelly Clamp |

Continued

Photo	Name	Construction and Functional Description	Nickname
	Crile	Serrations are full horizontal Straight and curved Length 5½" (14 cm) or 6¼" (15.9 cm)	Crile Clamp

	Rochester-Pean	Serrations are full horizontal Straight and curved (used to hold tissue flaps) Length 5½" (14 cm) to 12" (30.5 cm)	Pean-Mayo/ Mayo-Pean Clamp
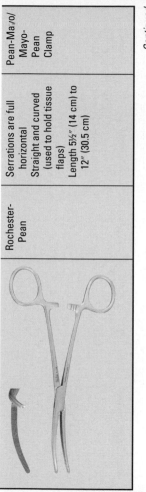			

Continued

Photo	Name	Construction and Functional Description	Nickname
	Rochester-Ochsner	Serrations are full horizontal Straight and curved, tips are 1 × 2 teeth (used to hold tissue and bone) Length 6¼″ (15.9 cm) to 10″ (25.4 cm)	Ochsner Mayo-Ochsner Clamp

Carmalt-Mayo/Carmal Clamp	Rochester-Carmalt		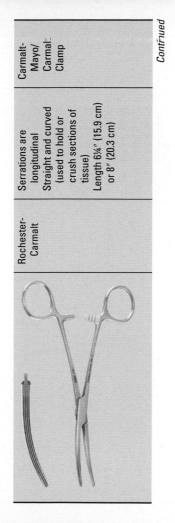
	Serrations are longitudinal Straight and curved (used to hold or crush sections of tissue) Length 6¼" (15.9 cm) or 8" (20.3 cm)		

Continued

Photo	Name	Construction and Functional Description	Nickname
Curved Straight	Curved and strait Ferguson Angiotribe forceps	Suitable for preventing and hemostasis of subsequent bleeding	

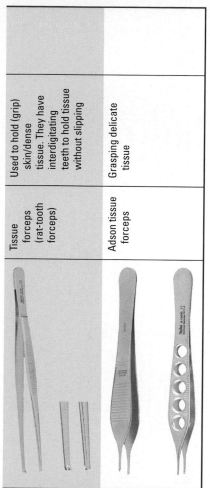

	Tissue forceps (rat-tooth forceps)	Used to hold (grip) skin/dense tissue. They have interdigitating teeth to hold tissue without slipping
	Adson tissue forceps	Grasping delicate tissue

Continued

Photo	Name	Construction and Functional Description	Nickname
	Brown-Adson tissue forceps	Multiple rows of teeth at a right angle, making them suitable for holding and manipulating subcutaneous tissue	
	Allis tissue forceps	Sharp teeth, used to hold or grasp heavy tissue	

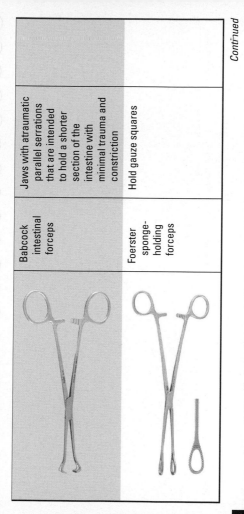

| | Babcock intestinal forceps | Jaws with atraumatic parallel serrations that are intended to hold a shorter section of the intestine with minimal trauma and constriction |
| | Foerster sponge-holding forceps | Hold gauze squares |

Continued

Photo	Name	Construction and Functional Description	Nickname
	Backhaus towel clamps	Hold towels	

	Jones towel clamp	Hold towels
	Grooved director	Aids both the fascial enlargement and closure
	Snook's ovariectomy hook	Used to retrieve the horn of the uterus while performing ovariohysterectomy

Continued

Photo	Name	Construction and Functional Description	Nickname
	Needle holders. (A) Derf (B) Olsen-Hegar (C) Mayo-Hegar	Grap needles	

Continued

	Metzenbaum scissors	Cutting delicate tissue	

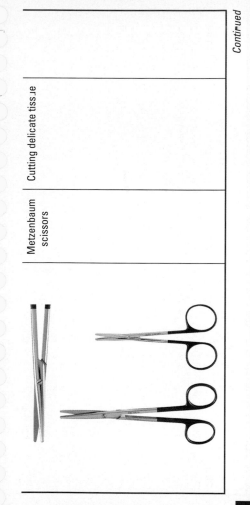

Photo	Name	Construction and Functional Description	Nickname
Straight Curved	Mayo scissors	Heavy scissors that can be straight or curved	Suture scissors

| | Operating scissors | Available in three tip configurations (sharp/sharp, blunt/blunt, or sharp/blunt), varying curvatures and multiple lengths, these scissors are used for general, multipurpose cutting and dissecting |

Sharp/sharp straight Sharp/blunt straight Blunt/blunt straight Sharp/sharp curved Sharp/blunt curved Blunt/blunt curved

Continued

Photo	Name	Construction and Functional Description	Nickname
	Wire scissors	Used to cut wire sutures in plastic and/or orthopedic surgery	
	Straight Spencer delicate-stitch scissors	Suture removal	Suture removal scissors

	Straight Littauer stitch scissors	Suture removal	Suture removal scissors
	Lister bandage scissors	Cutting bandages	Bandage scissors

Photo	Name	Construction and Functional Description	Nickname
	Knowles bandage scissors	Cutting bandages	
	Michel wound clip and applying forceps	Closing wounds	

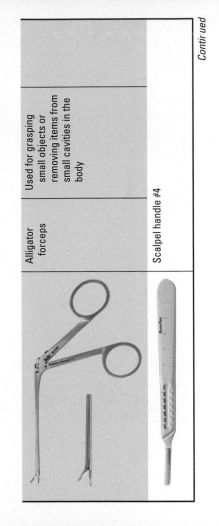

| | Alligator forceps | Used for grasping small objects or removing items from small cavities in the body | |
| | Scalpel handle #4 | | |

Continued

Photo	Name	Construction and Functional Description	Nickname
#10 #11 #12 #15	Scalpel blades.	#10—A general blade that is used for most procedures in small animals; fits a #3 handle. #11—Used to sever ligaments; fits a #3 handle. #12—Used to lance an abscess; fits a #3 handle. #15—Used for small, precise, or curved incisions	

SURGICAL PACK STORAGE[22]

Wrapper	Shelf Life
Double-wrapped, two-layer muslin	4 weeks
Double-wrapped, two-layer muslin, heat sealed in dust covers after sterilization	6 months
Double-wrapped, two-layer muslin, tape sealed in dust covers after sterilization	2 months
Double-wrapped nonwoven barrier materials (i.e., paper)	6 months
Paper/plastic peel pouches, heat sealed	1 year
Plastic peel pouches, heat sealed	1 year

PAIN EVALUATION[37]

SIGNS OF PAIN

Cardiovascular	Elevated heart rate and blood pressure, decreased peripheral circulation, prolonged capillary refill, cool extremities (ears, paws)
Respiratory	Rapid, shallow breaths, panting
Digestive	Weight loss, poor growth (young), vomiting, inappetence, constipation, diarrhea, salivation
Musculoskeletal	Unsteady gait, lameness, weakness, tremors, shivering
Urinary	Reluctance to urinate, loss of house training
Laboratory findings	Neutrophilia, lympho-cytosis, hyperglycemia, polycythemia, elevated cortisol, elevated catecholamines

PAIN EVALUATION

Signs of Pain	Suspected Pain Level	Duration
Head, Ear, Oral, Dental Surgery		
Rubbing; shaking; salivating; reluctance to eat, swallow, or drink; irritability, vocalizing	Moderate to high	Intermittent

Continued

Signs of Pain	Suspected Pain Level	Duration
Ophthalmologic		
Rubbing, vocalizing, reluctance to move	High	Intermittent to continual
Orthopedic		
Guarding, aggression, abnormal gait, self-mutilation, reluctance to move, dysuria, constipation	Moderate	Intermittent
Abdominal		
Guarding, splinting, abnormal posture, vomiting, inappetence	Mild to moderate	Intermittent
Cardiovascular/Thoracic		
Changes in respiratory rate and pattern, reluctance to move, vocalizing	Moderate to high	Continual
Perirectal		
Licking, biting, scooting, self-mutilation, constipation	Moderate	Intermittent

Dentistry

DIRECTIONAL TERMS USED IN DENTISTRY[9]

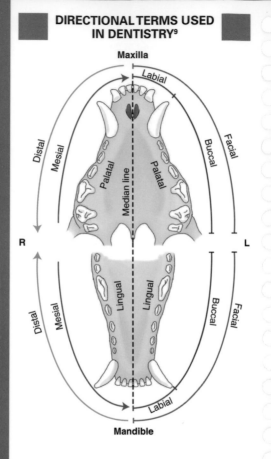

Maxilla

Labial

Facial

Distal

Mesial

Buccal

Palatal

Palatal

Median line

Maxilla

R

L

Distal

Mesial

Lingual

Lingual

Buccal

Facial

Labial

Mandible

COMMON DENTAL ABBREVIATIONS AND SYMBOLS FOR CHARTING THE MOUTH[52]

X	Extracted
0	Missing
FE F1 F2 F3	Furcation exposure Grade 1: furcation detected Grade 2: probe passes into furcation Grade 3: probe passes through furcation
RE	Root exposure
\	Tooth fracture
FXO	Open fracture
FXX	Closed fracture with no pulp evident
GH	Gingival hyperplasia
H	Gingival hyperplasia and then follow with the number to designate the millimeter of height
C	Calculus
C/H	Heavy calculus
C/M	Moderate calculus
C/S	Slight calculus
CLL	Cervical line lesion
CNL	Cervical neck lesion
FRL	Feline oral resorptive lesions
EH	Enamel hypocalcification (hypoplasia)
S	Supernumerary tooth

Continued

GR	Gingival recession—followed by number to designate millimeter decreased
M1	Slight mobility
M2	Moderate mobility: moderate tooth movement of 1 mm
M3	Severe mobility marked tooth movement of more than 1 mm
0	Health gingiva
I	Mild gingivitis with slight bleeding upon probing
II	Moderate gingivitis with edema or erythema and some bleeding
III	Severe gingivitis with swelling, pustular discharge, pocket formation, bleeding, and erythema

DENTAL DIRECTIONAL TERMS

Anodontia: All teeth are missing
Apical: Toward the apex (root)
Cementoenamel junction (CEJ): Area where the enamel and the cementum meet
Coronal: Toward the crown
Dens-in-dente: Enamel layer *folds* into itself or tooth
Dilacerated: Distorted (twisted) crown or root
Enamel hypocalcification ("hypoplasia"): Enamel pitting and/or discoloration
Enamel pearls: Beads of enamel at CEJ, furcation
Fusion tooth: Fusion of two tooth buds during formation

Gemination: Complete tooth duplication but incomplete split

godontia: Most teeth are missing

Hypodontia: Some teeth are missing

Interproximal: Surface between two teeth

Macrodontia: Oversized crown

Microdontia: Reduced crown

Mucogingival line (MGL): Junction of the attached gingival and mucosa

Occlusal: Surface of tooth facing a tooth in the opposite jaw

Subgingival: Below the gum line

Supernumerary: Extra tooth or teeth

Supragingival: Above the gum line

Twinning: Complete tooth duplication and split

DENTAL FORMULAS FOR CATS AND DOGS[52]

CATS

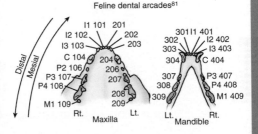

Feline dental arcades[81]

Deciduous (primary) teeth begin with the numbers 5, 6, 7, and 8

Deciduous: $2 \times (3i/3i, 1c/1c, PM3/3) = 26$

Permanent: $2 \times (3I/3I, 1C/1C, 3P/2P, 1M/1M) = 30$

Time of Eruption		
	Deciduous	**Permanent**
Incisors	2–3 weeks	3–4 months
Canines	3–4 weeks	4–5 months
Premolars	3–6 weeks	4–6 months
Molars		4–6 months

DOGS

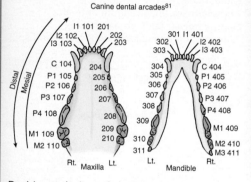

Canine dental arcades[81]

Deciduous (primary) teeth begin with the numbers 5, 6, 7, and 8

Deciduous: 2 × (3i/3i, 1c/1c, PM 3/3) = 28

Permanent: 2 × (3I/3I, 1C/1C, 4P/4P, 2M/3M) = 42

Time of Eruption		
	Deciduous	**Permanent**
Incisors	3–5 weeks	3–5 months
Canines	3–6 weeks	3.5–6 months
Premolars	4–10 weeks	3.5–6 months
Molars		3.5–7 months

NORMAL ROOT NUMBERS[29]

Numbers of roots in maxillary teeth of the dog

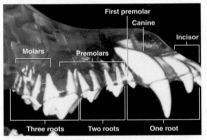

Numbers of roots in mandibular teeth of the dog

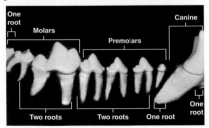

Number of roots in maxillary teeth of the cat

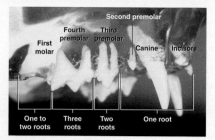

Numbers of roots in mandibular teeth of the cat

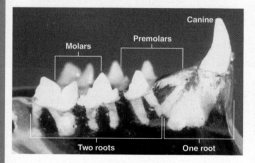

Parallel technique—Used for imaging of premolars and molars of mandible. The X-ray beam is directed from lateral to medial at right angles to the long axis of the tooth, which is parallel to the "film."

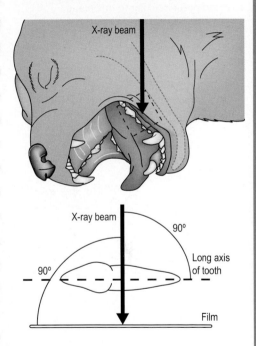

Bisecting angle technique—Used for imaging of incisors and canines of mandible and all maxillary teeth. An imaginary plane is drawn halfway between the plane of the film and a plane through the long axis of the tooth (the bisecting angle), and the X-ray beam is directed perpendicular to this plane.

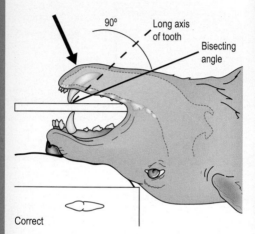

Tartar scrapers are single-ended and used to remove tartar and plaque from the surfaces of teeth.

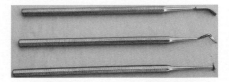

Jacquette tartar scalers are double-ended and used to remove tartar and plaque from the surfaces of teeth.

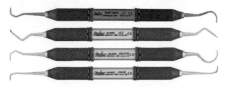

Columbia curettes are used to remove tartar from the subgingival surfaces of teeth.

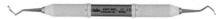

Dental explorers (A) and periodontal probes (B) are used to examine teeth for caries, calculi, furcations, and other abnormalities and to explore the depth of the sulci.

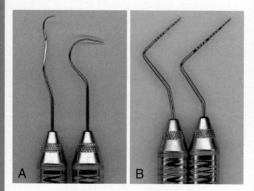

Tooth-splitting and separating forceps are used to split multirooted teeth for removal.

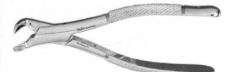

Incisor and root-extracting forceps grasp the small incisor or the root of a tooth that is to be removed.

Incisor-, canine-, and premolar-extracting forceps are used to remove incisor, canine, and premolar teeth.

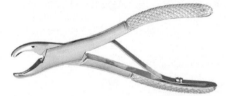

Dental elevators help loosen a tooth from the periodontal ligament before its extraction.

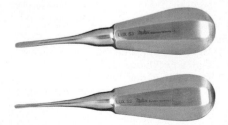

CLASSES OF RESORPTIVE LESIONS[52]

Description	Treatment
Stage 1	
Areas of erosion in the enamel	Use cavity varnish to seal dentinal tubules and harden enamel
Stage 2	
Lesions have penetrated the enamel and dentin	Restore with composite or glass ionomer cavity may varnish and only last 2 years
Stage 3	
Tooth has eroded into the endodontic system	Root canal with restoration; more likely tooth extraction
Stage 4	
Severe erosion apparent in crown and root structures	Extract tooth
Stage 5	
Crown is totally resorbed	No treatment unless area is inflamed, then extract root

Reasons to extract teeth

1. Generally any time there is a problem with a deciduous tooth
2. Retention of deciduous teeth
3. If mandibular/maxillary canines or incisors impinge or penetrate maxillary gingiva

4. Crowded teeth
5. Fractures with pulp exposure
6. Probing depth deeper than 5mm
7. Significant mobility
8. Roots with marked periapical lucency
9. Teeth with resorption causing inflammation
10. Radiographs reveal resorption
11. Marked chronic stomatitis
12. Grades 2 and 3 furcation

RECOMMENDATIONS AND PROTOCOLS

COMMON VACCINATIONS FOR DOGS[94A]

Vaccine Type	6-16 Weeks of Age	16 Weeks of Age and Older at the First Vaccination	Revaccination Within 1 Year of Last Vaccine	Revaccination After the First Year
Core Vaccines: Boosters Should Be 2-4 Weeks Apart				
DAPP or DHPP (MLV) • Canine distemper virus (also recombinant) • Parvovirus • Adenovirus-2, 6 • ±Parainfluenza virus	At least three doses of a combination vaccine	Two doses of a combination vaccine	A single dose	3 years
Rabies 1 year or 3 year (killed) Follow local law when applicable	As required by law			

Noncore Vaccines: Booster Should Be Recommended 2–4 Weeks Later for Some Dogs Based on Lifestyle, Geographic Location, and Risk of Exposure

Bordetella bronchiseptica and canine parainfluenza virus (intranasal)	One dose		One dose	One dose	Annually
B. bronchiseptica	Parenteral (SQ): Two initial doses IN: Single dose, Oral: Single dose		Parenteral (SQ): Two initial doses IN: Single dose Oral: Single dose	Single dose	Annually
Leptospira (killed) Serovars: Canicola, icterohaemorrhagiae, grippotyphosa, pomona	Two initial doses, as early as 12 weeks of age		Two initial doses	One dose	Annually

Continued

Vaccine Type	6–16 Weeks of Age	16 Weeks of Age and Older at the First Vaccination	Revaccination Within 1 Year of Last Vaccine	Revaccination After the First Year
Borrelia burgdorferi (canine Lyme disease) (killed and recombinant)	Two initial doses	Two initial doses	One dose	Annually
Canine influenza virus-H3N8 (killed)	Two initial doses	Two initial doses	One dose	Annually
Canine influenza virus-H3N2 (killed)	Two initial doses	Two initial doses	One dose	Annually
Crotalus atrox (Western Diamondback Rattlesnake)	Dosing requirements and frequency of administration vary among dogs depending on body weight and exposure risk			

COMMON VACCINES FOR CATS[95A]

Vaccine Type Follow Label Directions	Less Than 16 Weeks of Age When the First Dose Is Administered	Greater Than 16 Weeks of Age When the First Dose Is Administered	Revaccination
Core Vaccines			
Feline rhinotracheitis, calici and panleukopenia (HCP) and feline viral rhinotracheitis, calici, and panleukopenia (FVRCP)	No earlier than 6 weeks of age and then q3–4 weeks until 16–20 weeks of age	**Attenuated live:** One or two doses of a combination vaccine **Inactivated:** Two doses q3–4 weeks apart	Consider at 6 months* of age rather than 1 year to decrease the potential window of susceptibility if the kitten had maternally derived antibodies (MDA) and kitten booster at last
Feline herpesvirus (FHV)			Revaccinate q3 years thereafter
Feline calicivirus (FCV)		**Attenuated live intranasal:** One dose and then yearly thereafter	Revaccinate annually
Feline panleukopenia virus (FPV)			

Continued

Vaccine Type Follow Label Directions	Less Than 16 Weeks of Age When the First Dose Is Administered	Greater Than 16 Weeks of Age When the First Dose Is Administered	Revaccination
Feline leukemia virus (FeLV): Core vaccination under 1 year of age and high-risk cats over 1 year of age Noncore vaccine in cats that are low risk over 1 year of age Test to establish FeLV antigen status prior to vaccination	Test before vaccination Two doses 3–4 weeks apart beginning as early as 8 weeks of age	Two doses 3–4 weeks apart	**Inactivated vaccine:** Revaccinate 12 months after the last dose in the series then annually for individual cats at high risk of regular exposure through encountering FeLV+ cats, and cats of unknown FeLV status either indoors or outdoors

Recombinant (live canarypox vector): Revaccinate at 12 months after the last dose in the series and then consider revaccination:

- Annually for individual cats with regular exposure through living with FeLV+ cats and cats of unknown FeLV status either indoors or outdoors
- Every 2–3 years, where product licensure allows, for individual adult cats less likely to have regular exposure to FeLV+ cats

Continued

Vaccine Type Follow Label Directions	Less Than 16 Weeks of Age When the First Dose Is Administered	Greater Than 16 Weeks of Age When the First Dose Is Administered	Revaccination
			NOTE: At-risk (fighting, outdoor lifestyle, etc.) adult cats should continue to be vaccinated against FeLV annually. Revaccinate every 2 years in periodic exposure situations in mature cats. Where vaccines with a 3-year duration of immunity are available, their use can be considered

	Follow local laws	Follow local laws	Recommended when the law is applicable: 3-year vaccination interval using a 3-year labeled vaccine
Rabies (recombinant and inactivated)			
Noncore Vaccines			
Chlamydophila felis: Chlamydia (attenuated live and inactivated and **parenteral**)	For frequency and interval, follow label instructions		
B. bronchiseptica (attenuated live **intranasal**)	For frequency and interval, follow label instructions		

RETROVIRAL TESTING RECOMMENDATIONS IN CATS[96A]

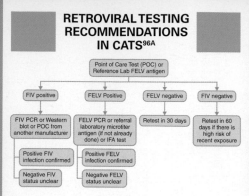

Point of Care Test (POC) or Reference Lab FELV antigen

FIV positive
- FIV PCR or Western blot or POC from another manufacturer
  - Positive FIV infection confirmed
  - Negative FIV status unclear

FELV Positive
- FELV PCR or referral laboratory microtiter antigen (if not already done) or IFA test
  - Positive FELV infection confirmed
  - Negative FELV status unclear

FELV negative
- Retest in 30 days

FIV negative
- Retest in 60 days if there is high risk of recent exposure

Note: Cats that have been vaccinated for FIV will test positive.

VETORYL TREATMENT AND MONITORING FLOWCHART[97]

Treatment and Monitoring of Hyperadrenocorticism

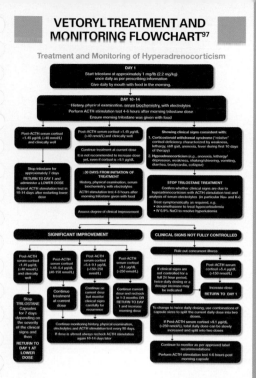

DAY 1
Start trilostane at approximately 1 mg/lb (2.2 mg/kg)
once daily as per prescribing information
Give daily by mouth with food in the morning.

DAY 10-14
History, physical examination, serum biochemistry, with electrolytes
Perform ACTH stimulation test 4-6 hours after morning trilostane dose
Ensure morning trilostane was given with food

Post-ACTH serum cortisol <1.45 μg/dL (<40 nmol/L) and clinically well

Post-ACTH serum cortisol >1.45 μg/dL (>40 nmol/L) and clinically well

Continue treatment at current dose
It is not recommended to increase dose yet, even if cortisol is >9.1 μg/dL

Stop trilostane for approximately 7 days
RETURN TO DAY 1 and administer a LOWER DOSE
Repeat ACTH stimulation test in 10-14 days after restarting lower dose

≥30 DAYS FROM INITIATION OF TREATMENT
History, physical examination, serum biochemistry, with electrolytes
ACTH stimulation test 4-6 hours after morning trilostane given with food

Assess degree of clinical improvement

Showing clinical signs consistent with:
1. Corticosteroid withdrawal syndrome ("relative" cortisol deficiency characterized by weakness, lethargy, stiff gait, anorexia, fever during first 10 days of therapy)
2. Hypoadrenocorticism (e.g., anorexia, lethargy/ depression, weakness, shaking/shivering, vomiting, diarrhea, bradycardia, collapse)

STOP TRILOSTANE TREATMENT
Confirm whether clinical signs are due to hypoadrenocorticism with ACTH stimulation test and analysis of serum electrolytes (in particular Na+ and K+)
Treat symptomatically as required, e.g.
• dexamethasone to treat hypocortisolemia
• IV 0.9% NaCl to resolve hyperkalemia

SIGNIFICANT IMPROVEMENT

Post-ACTH serum cortisol <1.45 μg/dL (<40 nmol/L) and clinically well

Post-ACTH serum cortisol 1.45-5.4 μg/dL (40-150 nmol/L)

Post-ACTH serum cortisol >5.4-9.1 μg/dL (>150-250 nmol/L)

Post-ACTH serum cortisol >9.1 μg/dL (>250 nmol/L)

Stop TRILOSTANE Capsules for 7 days depending on the severity of the clinical signs and then RETURN TO DAY 1 AT LOWER DOSE

Continue treatment at current dose

Continue on current dose but monitor clinical signs carefully for recurrence

Continue current dose and recheck in 1-3 months OR RETURN TO DAY 1 and increase dosing

Continue monitoring history, physical examination, electrolytes and ACTH stimulation test every 90 days.
If dose is altered always recheck ACTH stimulation again 10-14 days later

CLINICAL SIGNS NOT FULLY CONTROLLED

Rule out concurrent illness

If clinical signs are not controlled for a full 24 hour period, twice daily dosing or a dosage increase may be indicated

Post-ACTH serum cortisol >5.4 μg/dL (>150 nmol/L)

Increase dose
RETURN TO DAY 1

To change to twice daily dosing, use combinations of capsule sizes to split the current daily dose into two doses.
If Post-ACTH serum cortisol >9.1 μg/dL (>250 nmol/L), total daily dose can be slowly increased and split into two doses

Continue to monitor as per approved label recommendations
Perform ACTH stimulation test 4-6 hours post morning capsule

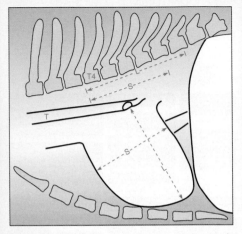

Buchanan JW, Bucheler J: Vertebral scale system to measure canine heart size in radiographs, *J AM Vet Med Assoc* 206: 194, 1995.

Diagram illustrates the vertebral heart score (VHS) measurement method using the lateral chest radiograph. The long-axis (L) and short-axis (S) heart dimensions are transposed onto the vertebral column and recorded as the number of vertebrae beginning with the cranial edge of T4. These values are added to obtain the VHS. In this example, L = 5.8 v, S = 4.6 v, therefore VHS = 10.4 v. *T,* Trachea.

SOURCES

An "A" in the reference citation indicates that material was adapted from the source cited.

1. Ackerman N: *Aspinall's complete textbook of veterinary nursing*, ed 3, Edinburgh, Scotland, 2016, Elsevier Ltd.
2. Aspinall V: *Clinical procedures in veterinary nursing*, ed 3, Edinburgh, Scotland, 2014, Butterworth-Heinemann.
3. Bassert JM, Beal AD, Samples OM: *McCurnin's clinical textbook for veterinary technicians*, ed 9, St. Louis, 2018, Elsevier.
4. Bassert JM, Thomas JA: *McCurnin's clinical textbook for veterinary technicians*, ed 8, St. Louis, 2014, Saunders.
5. Battaglia A, Steele A: *Small animal emergency and critical care for veterinary technicians*, ed 3, St. Louis, 2016, Elsevier.
6. Battaglia A: *Small animal emergency and critical care*, ed 2, St. Louis, 2007, Elsevier.
7. Bill RL: *Clinical pharmacology and therapeutics for veterinary technicians*, ed 4, St. Louis, 2017, Elsevier.
8. Bowman DD: *Georgis' parasitology for veterinarians*, ed 10, St. Louis, 2014, Saunders.
9. Brown M, Brown L: *Lavin's radiography for veterinary technicians*, ed 5, St. Louis, 2013, Saunders.
10. Brunzel NA: *Fundamentals of urine and body fluid analysis*, ed 4, St. Louis, 2018, Elsevier.
11. Busch SJ: *Small animal surgical nursing: skills and concepts*, St. Louis, 2006, Elsevier.
12. Chew DJ, DiBartola SP, Schenck PA: *Canine and feline nephrology and urology*, ed 2, St. Louis, 2011, Saunders.
13. Colville T, Bassert JM: *Clinical anatomy and physiology for veterinary technicians*, ed 3, St. Louis, 2016, Elsevier.
14. Copyright © Royal Canin SAS.
15. Côté E: *Clinical vet advisor: dogs and cats*, St. Louis, 2007, Saunders.
16. Cowell RL, Rick L: *Diagnostic cytology and hematology of the dog and cat*, ed 3, St. Louis, 2008, Mosby.
17. Cowell RL, Tyler RD, Meinkoth JH: *Diagnostic cytology and hematology of the dog and cat*, ed 2, St. Louis, 1999, Mosby.
18. Cowell RL, Valenciano AC: *Cowell and Tyler's diagnostic cytology and hematology of the dog and cat*, ed 4, St. Louis, 2014, Mosby.

19. Edwards NJ: *ECG manual for the veterinary technician,* St. Louis, 1993, Saunders.

20. Feldman EC, Ettinger SJ: *Textbook of veterinary internal medicine,* ed 7, St. Louis, 2010, Saunders.

21. Ford F, Mazzaferro E: *Kirk and Bistner's handbook of veterinary procedures and emergency treatment,* ed 8, St. Louis, 2006, Saunders.

22. Fossum TW, editor: *Small animal surgery,* ed 3, St. Louis, 2007, Mosby.

23. Gorrel C: *Veterinary dentistry for the general practitioner,* ed 2, Edinburgh, Scotland, 2013, Elsevier Ltd.

24. Han C, Hurd C: *Practical diagnostic imaging for the veterinary technician,* ed 3, St. Louis, 2003, Mosby.

25. Harvey JW: *Veterinary hematology,* St. Louis, 2012, Saunders.

26. Harvey JW, editor: *Veterinary hematology,* St. Louis, 2012, Saunders. Courtesy of DE Brown and MA Thrall

27. Hendrix CM, Robinson E: *Diagnostic parasitology for veterinary technicians,* ed 3, St. Louis, 2006, Mosby.

28. Hendrix CM, Sirois M: *Laboratory procedures for veterinary technicians,* ed 5, St. Louis, 2007, Mosby.

29. Holmstrom S: *Veterinary dentistry for the technician and office staff,* St. Louis, 2000, Saunders.

30. Jorgensen Laboratories, Inc. Loveland, Colorado.

31. Kumar V, Abbas AK, Aster JC, editors: *Robbins basic pathology,* ed 9, St. Louis, 2013, Saunders.

32. Little S: *The cat: clinical medicine and management,* St. Louis, 2012, Saunders.

33. Maggs DJ, Miller PE, Ofri R: *Slatter's fundamentals of veterinary ophthalmology,* ed 4, St. Louis, 2008, Saunders.

34. Marks SL, Willard MD: Diarrhea in kittens. In August JR, editor: *Consultations in feline internal medicine,* ed 5, St. Louis, 2006, Saunders Elsevier, pp 136.

35. McBride DF: *Learning veterinary terminology,* ed 2, St. Louis, 2002, Mosby.

36. McCurnin DM, Bassert JM: *Clinical textbook for veterinary technicians,* ed 5, St. Louis, 2002, Saunders.

37. McCurnin DM, Bassert JM: *Clinical textbook for veterinary technicians,* ed 6, St. Louis, 2006, Saunders.

38. McCurnin DM, Bassert JM: *McCurnin's clinical textbook for veterinary technicians,* ed 7, St. Louis, 2010, Saunders.

39. McCurnin DM, Poffenbarger EM: *Small animal physical diagnosis and clinical procedures,* St. Louis, 1991, WB Saunders.

40. McKelvey D, Hollingsworth KW: *Veterinary anesthesia and analgesics,* ed 3, St. Louis, 2003, Mosby.

41. Miller WH, Griffin CE, Campbell KL: *Muller and Kirk's small animal dermatology*, ed 7, St. Louis, 2013, Mosby.

42. Levine D, Millis DL. *Canine rehabilitation and physical therapy*, ed 2, St. Louis, 2014, Saunders.

43. Nemitz R: *Surgical instrumentation: an interactive approach*, St. Louis, 2009, WB Saunders.

44. Permission granted by Integra LifeSciences Corporation, Plainsboro, New Jersey, USA.

45. Peterson ME, Kutzler MA; *Small animal pediatrics*, St. Louis, 2011, Saunders.

46. Raskin RE, Meyer DJ: *Atlas of canine and feline cytology*, St. Louis, 2001, Saunders.

47. Raskin RE, Meyer DJ, editors: *Canine and feline cytology*, ed 2, St. Louis, 2010, Saunders.

48. Raskin RE, Meyer DJ, editors: *Canine and feline cytology*, ed 2, St. Louis, 2010, Saunders. Courtesy of Rose Raskin, University of Florida.

49. Raskin RE, Meyer DJ, editors: *Canine and feline cytology*, ed 3, St. Louis, 2016, Elsevier.

50. Sheldon CC, Sonsthagen TF, Topel JA: *Animal restraint for veterinary professionals*, ed 2, St. Louis, 2017, Elsevier.

51. Sirois M: *Laboratory procedures for veterinary technicians*, ed 6, St. Louis, 2015, Mosby.

52. Sirois M: *Principles and practice of veterinary technology*, ed 2, St. Louis, 2004, Mosby.

53. Sirois M: *Principles and practice of veterinary technology*, ed 3, St. Louis, 2011, Mosby.

54. Sirois M: *Principles and practice of veterinary technology*, ed 4, St. Louis, 2017, Elsevier.

55. Songer JG, Post KW: *Veterinary microbiology: bacterial and fungal agents of animal disease*, St. Louis, 2005, Saunders.

56. Sonsthagen T: *Veterinary instruments and equipment: a pocket guide*, ed 3, St. Louis, 2014, Mosby.

57. Taylor SM: *Small animal clinical techniques*, ed 2, St. Louis, 2016, Elsevier.

58. Taylor SM, editor: *Small animal clinical techniques*, ed 2, St. Louis, 2016, Elsevier. Courtesy of Dr. Klaas Post, University of Saskatchewan.

59. Tear M: *Small animal surgical nursing*, ed 3, St. Louis, 2017, Elsevier.

60. Tear M: *Small animal surgical nursing*, ed 3, St. Louis, 2017, Elsevier. Photo by John T. Miller.

61. Thomas JA, Lerche P: *Anesthesia and analgesia for veterinary technicians*, ed 5, St. Louis, 2017, Elsevier.

62. Tighe MM, Brown M: *Mosby's comprehensive review for veterinary technicians*, ed 4, St. Louis, 2015, Mosby.

63. Willard MD, Tvedten H: *Small animal clinical diagnosis by laboratory methods*, ed 5, St. Louis, 2012, Saunders.

64. Peterson M, Talcott PA: *Small animal toxicology*, ed 3, St. Louis, 2013, Elsevier.

65. Geor R: *Equine sports medicine and surgery: basic and clinical sciences of the equine athlete*, ed 2, St. Louis, 2014, Elsevier.

66. Cohn L: *Côté's clinical veterinary advisor: dogs and cats*, ed 4, St. Louis, 2020, Elsevier.

67. El-Hussein MT: *Huether and McCance's understanding pathophysiology*, Second Canadian Edition, 2023.

68. McGavin MD: *Pathologic basis of veterinary disease*, ed 4, 2007.

69. Thomson C: *Veterinary neuroanatomy: a clinical approach*, 2012.

70. Nelson RW, Guillermo Couto C, editors: *Small animal internal medicine*, ed 5, St. Louis, 2014, Elsevier.

71. Auerbach A: *Diagnostic pathology: spleen*, ed 2, 2022.

72. Beal AD, Bassert JM, Samples OM: *McCurnin's clinical textbook for veterinary technicians and nurses*, ed 10, St. Louis, 2022, Elsevier.

73. Patricia M: *Tille, Bailey & Scott's diagnostic microbiology*, ed 15, St. Louis, 2022, Elsevier.

74. Rifai N: *Tietz textbook of clinical chemistry and molecular diagnostics*, ed 6, Philadelphia, 2018, Saunders.

75. Bassert J: *McCurnin's clinical textbook for veterinary technicians and nurses*, ed 10, Philadelphia, 2022, Saunders.

76. Sirois M: *Laboratory procedures for veterinary technicians*, ed 7, St. Louis, 2020, Mosby.

77. Pedigo RA, Kaji A: *Emergency medicine board review*, St. Louis, 2022, Elsevier.

78. Bolognia J, Schaffer J, Duncan K, Ko C, editors: *Dermatology essentials*, ed 2, St. Louis, 2022, Elsevier.

79. Malamed S: *Medical emergencies in the dental office*, ed 8, St. Louis, 2023, Elsevier.

80. Kruger R, Anthony J, Frownfelter D, Dean E, Stout M: *Cardiovascular and pulmonary physical therapy: evidence to practice*, ed 6, St. Louis, 2023, Elsevier.

81. Christenson DE: *Veterinary medical terminology*, ed 3, St. Louis, 2020, Elsevier.

82. Gay CC, Hinchcliff KW, Studdert VP: *Saunders comprehensive veterinary dictionary*, ed 5, St. Louis, 2021, Elsevier.

83. Chabot-Richards D, Foucar K, Karner KH, Czuchlewski DR, Vasef MA, Reichard KK, Zhang QY, Wilson CS,

Culbreath K: *Diagnostic pathology: blood and bone marrow*, ed 2, St. Louis, 2018, Elsevier.

84. Bhattacharya GK: *Concise pathology for exam preparation*, ed 4, St. Louis, 2021, Elsevier.

85. Raskin RE, Meyer DJ, Boes KM: *Canine and feline cytopathology: a color atlas and interpretation guide*, ed 4, St. Louis, 2023, Elsevier.

86. Gaynor JS, Muir MW: *Handbook of veterinary pain management*, St. Louis, 2002, Elsevier, pp 152–156, 210–230, 407–410.

87. Paddleford RR: *Manual of small animal anesthesia*, ed 2, Philadelphia, 1999, Saunders, pp 19–24.

88. Stein B., Thompson D., et al.: *Analgesic constant rate infusions*, Veterinary Anesthesia & Analgesia Support Group, October 2005. http://www.vasg.org/constant_rate_infusions.htm (edited 11–11).

89. Cassarino D: *Diagnostic pathology: neoplastic dermatopathology*, ed 3, St. Louis, 2022, Elsevier.

90. Cowell RL, Valenciano AC: *Cowell and Tyler's diagnostic cytology and hematology of the dog and cat*, ed 5, St. Louis, 2020, Elsevier.

91. Adapted from The VSPN Notebook®. ©Veterinary Information Network®.

92. Table contents sourced from the Companion Animal Parasite Council General Guidelines, https://capcvet.org/guidelines/general-guidelines.

93. American Heartworm Society, 2020_AHS_Canine_Guidelines_Summary_11_12.pdf.

94. American Animal Hospital Association (AAHA): 2022 AAHA Canine Vaccination Guidelines, https://doi.org/10.5326/JAAHA-MS-Canine-Vaccination-Guidelines.

95. AAHA and American Association of Feline Practitioners (AAFP): 2020 AAHA/AAFP Feline Vaccination Guidelines, https://catvets.com/guidelines/practice-guidelines/aafp-aaha-feline-vaccination.

96. Little S, Levy J, Hartmann K, Lehmann RH, Hosle M, Olah G, Denis KS: 2020 AAFP feline retrovirus testing and management guidelines, *J Feline Med Surg* 22: 5–30, 2020. Sage ©ISFM and AAFP 2020, https://journals.sagepub.com/doi/pdf/10.1177/1098612X19895940.

97. © 2023 Dechra Veterinary Products LLC and/or its affiliates. All rights reserved.

98. Veterinary Teaching Hospital, Colorado State University, http://www.cvmbs.colostate.edu/clinsci/wing/fluids/cri.htm.

99. American College of Veterinary Surgeons (ACVS), http://www.acvs.org/symposium/proceedings2011/data/papers/157.pdf.

100. Zachary JF: *Pathologic basis of veterinary disease*, ed 7, St. Louis, 2022, Elsevier.

101. Courtesy of Dr. T. Olivry, College of Veterinary Medicine, North Carolina State University.

102. Johnston SA, Tobias KM: *Veterinary surgery: small animal*, ed 2, St. Louis, 2018, Elsevier.

103. Hnilica K: *Small animal dermatology*, ed 3, St. Louis, 2011, Saunders.

104. Fossum TW, editor: *Small animal surgery*, ed 4, St. Louis, 2013, Elsevier.

105. Brunzel NA: *Fundamentals of urine and body fluid analysis*, ed 5, St. Louis, 2023, Elsevier.

106. Hnilica KA, Patterson A: *Small animal dermatology: a color atlas and therapeutic guide*, ed 4, St. Louis, 2017, Saunders.

107. From Adachi JA, Backer HD, DuPont HL: Infectious diarrhea from wilderness and foreign travel. In Auerbach PS, Cushing TA, Harris NS, editors: *Auerbach's wilderness medicine* ed 7, St. Louis, 2017, Elsevier, pp. 1859–1874, Fig. 82.2.

108. With permission from Taplin D, Meinking TL: Infestations. In Schachner LA, Hansen RC, editors: *Pediatric dermatology* ed 4. Edinburgh, Scotland, 2011, Mosby, pp. 1141–1180.

109. Modified from Cho J: Surgery of the globe and orbit, *Top Companion Anim Med* 23(23), 2008.

110. Kradin RL: *Diagnostic pathology of infectious disease*, St. Louis, 2010, Elsevier.

111. Courtesy Francisco Conrado, University of Florida. Raskin, RE, Meyer, DJ, Boes, KM: *Canine and feline cytopathology: a color atlas and interpretation guide*, ed 4, St. Louis, 2023, Elsevier.

112. Buchanan JW, Bucheler J: Vertebral scale system to measure canine heart size in radiographs, *J AM Vet Med Assoc* 206: 194, 1995.

Note: Page numbers followed by "*f*" indicate figures, "*t*" indicate tables, and "*b*" indicate boxes.

423

Veterinary PDQ

Kristin Holtgrew-Bohling, DVM

Get quick access to the information a vet tech needs every day!

Ideal for the clinical setting, this full-color guide covers key topics such as the physical exam, common diseases, emergency care, pharmacology, diagnostic procedures and imaging techniques, surgery and anesthesia, parasite identification, blood tests, and other lab work—in short, all the information that is most useful in practice.

OUTSTANDING FEATURES:

- **NEW!** Updated drug information includes the newest pharmacologic agents and their uses, dosage forms, and adverse side effects.
- Valuable formulas, conversions, and lab values make it easy to look up data.
- Easy-to-read charts and tables summarize important information that vet techs commonly use but rarely memorize.
- Full-color photos and drawings illustrate procedures and tests, dental and surgical instruments, parasites, and urine and blood analysis.
- Spiral binding allows you to lay the book flat or keep it open to a specific page, and durable pages can withstand everyday use.

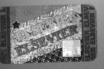

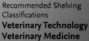

Recommended Shelving
Classifications
Veterinary Technology
Veterinary Medicine

ISBN 978-0-323-88149-4

9 780323 881494

ELSEVIER